Eat Like You Teach

EAT LIKE YOU TEACH

How to Reset Your Weight *and* Reclaim Your Life

IRENE PACE, RD

M·J

NEW YORK

LONDON • NASHVILLE • MELBOURNE • VANCOUVER

EAT LIKE YOU TEACH

How to Reset Your Weight and Reclaim Your Life

Published in New York, New York, by Morgan James Publishing in partnership with Difference Press. Morgan James is a trademark of Morgan James, LLC.
www.MorganJamesPublishing.com

ISBN 9781642796896 paperback
ISBN 9781642796902 eBook
Library of Congress Control Number: 2019943714

Cover Design by:
Megan Dillon
megan@creativeninjadesigns.com

Interior Design by:
Chris Treccani
www.3dogcreative.net

Emotions Wheel graphic by Geoffrey Roberts
All other graphics by W.T.L.Rathnasekara

For my children Lacey, Daphne, and Hugh who engaged in the most creative and entertaining self-directed play while I wrote. I love you guys like crazy. My world is an infinitely better place with you in it.

For Bose who makes the best noise cancelling headphones on the market.

Table of Contents

Chapter 1:
An Introduction

"I don't have to know how to solve a problem in me. I just have to be willing to have a new experience. Practice observing. Practice acceptance. Practice willingness."
–Tracy McMillian

Being a nutrition professional who is struggling with eating sucks. It's not just about your pants not fitting or the mind games you play with yourself like you can almost feel your arteries slamming shut (true story) or it's somehow okay because what you're impulsively eating is fruit and cottage cheese (also a true story). It's isolating, distracting, and it messes with your confidence, your identity, and your integrity. You don't turn to friends for support because you're their go-to for all things nutrition. Outing yourself to colleagues feels like career suicide (not to mention more shame than you could bear right now).

As your waistline grows, you feel like it's the elephant in the room. You're distracted in appointments, wondering if your clients are onto you. The word "fraud" invades your thoughts like that song you can't stand but can't get out of your head. Eating trouble is not only costing you your health and eroding your confidence, but it's beginning to pick away at your sanity too.

I bet you've tried to figure this out. Maybe casually at first when you felt a little off-track. You tightened things up for a while. At some point you thought, "Okay, I better *do* something about this. Time to get serious." Perhaps that looked like a highly detailed meal plan and tracking sheet or apps or both. Perhaps you went the route of expertly calculated macros and meal templates (but which ratios to use… hmmm?). Perhaps, even though you *know* it never works, you said goodbye to bread or chocolate or cheese "forever."

What would you give right now to have your eating back on track? To go to bed at night knowing you've got this (and your pants will fit in the morning)? To feel sharp and focused at work and enjoy time with your family and friends - free from the weight of this secret you've been hauling around?

This book serves to help you reset and experience what it feels like to get your eating back in alignment with your values and your identity. To put an end to creeping weight and the worry that goes along with watching your waistline grow. To let you know that you're not alone and to give you a clear plan from a trusted source to get back to living life the way that matters most to you.

Invite All Parts of You Along for the Ride

Parts of you want to show up in the biggest of ways and do what you know needs to be done to see yourself through this. Other parts of you are afraid. What is this is going to look like? What if it doesn't work? What if you actually *are* a fraud? What if you're doomed to just keep eating like this and gaining weight and feeling like crap forever?

While I can't take your fear away, I *can* tell the part of you that is afraid this: I had the same fears and it's ok to be afraid and do it anyway. It *will* be difficult but *so* worth it. The tools and system I share with you here are the ones I use to help myself and others like you. Every. Single. Day. One sure thing is that time will tick forward. You can pass that time continuing to do what you already know isn't working *or* you can try a different way. What you're doing now will always be there to go back to - anytime you choose.

Feeling conflicted is a normal, and even necessary, part of the change process. You know this and you see it in your clients *all the time*. It's *different* when it happens to you, right? It is, but it isn't. The question becomes, how can you feel conflicted and move forward anyway?

Let the part of you that wants to keep reading, help the part of you that is afraid. It's not exactly *that* easy, but the solution is a lot less complicated than you allow yourself to believe. It seems fitting that a big messy problem should have an equally complicated solution, right? I thought so, too.

Here's what I learned instead.

The Small, Less Complicated Solution

Consistent and persistent actions trump big grand gestures. It's the small actions that you take every day, every hour, every moment, that matter most. No choice is neutral. Each choice moves you towards or away from where you want to go and who you want to be. There is huge opportunity in that. Any moment is a chance to begin again. You get to cast little votes in favor of you over and over and over. The end game is to be consistent and persistent at taking actions that are best for your body, and your life. To, most of the time, choose the actions that serve you best.

If you're still here reading, I imagine you want to know how to do that. Welcome to my story and the strategies that changed my life. The principles in this book have the power to change your life too. You will see more clearly where you keep getting stuck. You will know a way though this is possible if you are willing to think differently and lean into discovering and following a path that is uniquely yours.

To begin, you get to figure out what works for you. What is best for you and your body and your life. In order to take consistent and persistent action on something, you have to know what that something is. You can't figure this one out in your head, sorry think-y folks. You've got to try stuff. Get open to, and deliberate about, experiencing new things. I'll teach you a system to do just that.

Next, once you find what works for you, get consistent and persistent about doing it. You'll explore what helps you be more consistent and how to do more of that. You'll look at what gets in the way of you being consistent and how can you clear those obstacles from your path.

In Part I: Reality (Chapters two and three) you'll get a deeper look at the solution and learn about building an Owner's Manual for yourself. A set of handling instructions for your body and your life that open the door for you to care for yourself like someone you are responsible for caring for.

In Part II: Reboot (Chapters four to six) you will learn principles and a framework to figure stuff out and build your Owner's Manual.

In Part III: Reset (Chapters seven to nine) you put that framework into action to build the Eating, Movement, Sleep, and Environment sections of your Owner's Manual.

In Part IV: Reclaim (Chapters ten to twelve) you'll learn strategies to get consistent and persistent and put the Owner's Manual you just created into action, no matter what life throws your way.

This book is about helping you back to what matters to you. It's about discovering and owning what works for your body and your life, no matter what anyone else thinks or believes or does. It's about moving from knowing to doing and then from doing to doing consistently. Trading big grand temporary gestures for every day actions, votes in favor of you, that move you in the direction of your desired future self.

Part I:

Reality

Chapter 2:

Be Human – Like You Have a Choice

"Are you gonna cry about it or boss up? First of all imma do both."
- Unknown

As my therapy session was wrapping up, I was real-time processing the massive spread of things we had just covered.

We all grapple with the same big fat hairy life questions:

"Am I worthy? Am I good enough?"

"Will this work?"

"What if I'm actually broken, weird, or doomed in some way?"

I think we touched on all three of those that day. It was a teary session for me. Not a full-on, ugly-cry jam but teary enough that I was grateful to be wearing waterproof mascara.

After spending the first part of the session exploring the almighty topic of worthiness, Dr. E. gracefully guided me through dissecting my long list of "shoulds." His skillful questions put on display the ridiculous expectations I have for myself, how they are not serving me, and how the logic I construct behind them is faulty *but*, at the same time, also makes sense.

As I finished wiping my streaky face and packed away my notebook, I looked at him with a cheeky half smile and said, "Well, isn't this fantastic. I get to feel worthless *and* expect extraordinary things from myself all at the same time." He smiled back warmly and said, "The inconveniences of being human."

2015 was the beginning of a time of massive personal growth for me. I had just gone back to work after a decade being mostly home with my three young kids. My stress level was high and my time for self-care was low. When I found myself struggling with food, it was the last straw. It was such a blow to my identity to have my eating feel out of control, to barely fit into the maternity jeans I secretly pulled out again (stretch panel to the rescue), to spend my days helping clients through their eating challenges only to come home and watch myself struggle with those same things.

It was my shameful little secret until my expanding waistline threatened to out me. I would rally and have a few "perfect" days and then fall back into old habits. Again, a cycle I help coach clients through *all* the time. At some point along the way, I would get sick of the white-knuckling and just take my hands off the wheel.

I struggled alone because I didn't want to admit I was a dietitian who needed help with her eating. I felt like a fraud. I worried that it wouldn't be long before others would know – especially if I couldn't stop my weight from creeping up. I finally came to the conclusion I had to do something *different*. Since I was basically hiding from the world (and from myself) that I needed nutrition help, I invested in the next best thing that made sense. I hired a personal trainer, and I hit the gym – hard. It didn't solve my eating woes, but looking back, it was a significant step on the path that led me here. It taught me these important lessons:

1. Trying harder at what is not working will never work.
2. Experiences have a way of leading you to solutions you could never think your way to.

Even when you aren't clear on what else to do, continuing to do the same thing you *know* is not working makes no logical sense. Yet we all do it, right? Do the same thing, and hope for a different result. Favour the familiarity of the broken thing you know over the fear of the unknown. The trouble with this is twofold. First, time doesn't wait, and you continue further along the *not working* path. Which is usually not great, or it wouldn't be a problem in the first place. Second, no exposure to new experiences means no exposure to possible new solutions.

Phillip McKernan, a coach of mine, says, "In the absence of clarity, take action." While you're waiting for the answer or clarity to emerge, do something else. Try something new, anything new. Glean from the experiences of others who have walked a similar path before you (good on you for grabbing this book, right?). Then try something. Be a gatherer of new experiences. See what works for you. Repeat.

Taking *some* action (hiring a trainer) prompted a whole bunch of other actions in me that eventually showed me what I needed to figure this out. I started reading more self-help books and listening to podcasts. Courses, workshops, certifications, and personal development events made their way on to my calendar. I stumbled across an online nutrition company named Precision Nutrition (PN). When I found their philosophy aligned beautifully with mine, I registered for their Level 1 certification course and plugged into their groups and networks. Connecting with a community full of like-minded, caring folks was another significant step on my path.

While doing the course, I learned about PN's online nutrition coaching program. I knew I was struggling with my eating, but the thought about getting *myself* a *nutrition* coach had never crossed my mind. I mean, how could I justify that? I'm an R.D. for Pete's sake. I know exactly what to do to get a few pounds off and get back on track. I'm just not doing it. On registration day, I had an overwhelming sense that I had to go for it. I had to invest in me.

In July 2016, I signed on to work with a nutrition coach. Yup, me, a dietitian who knows all the things and helps others with their eating every day, signed up with a coach. I told myself it was an "empathy exercise" to be on the client side of the table (wasn't that nice of me to frame it that way for myself?) My year as Coach Pam's client challenged and changed me in ways I could not have imagined. I finished the year at the same weight I started. My desired physical changes would come later, but the change that happened *inside* me that year was off the charts. I continued to pursue personal and professional growth in every way possible. My fear of being the coach with a coach was gone. When I got stuck at something, I got help. Do I think I would have figured this nutrition piece out on my own? Maybe. Eventually. But all the other stuff I learned along the way has been priceless, and I can't imagine where I'd be if I had missed that experience. If there is ever a chance I can fast-track my way through a mess that impacts my life, I'm going to choose that. Life is too short and too precious not to.

I experienced the power a skilled coach had to evoke change in me. I finally accepted and embraced that change can only come through discomfort (and sometimes pain). Discomfort is not only likely in the change process; it's essential. That makes sense, right? If you are comfortable in something or tolerate it even if you don't like it, there is not enough pressure to move you to change it. Change becomes inevitable when the pain of staying where you are is greater than the pain of making the change. If you're here reading this book, I'm guessing you may be there. Ray Dalio's book *Principles* is full of valuable insights including this one: Principle 2.2 A, "View painful problems as potential improvements that are screaming at you." There was a lot of screaming, and I answered the call.

On the professional front, I was able to help my clients in new ways. I had a truckload of new tools to help them get unstuck in places I couldn't before, and it felt fantastic. As I reflected on my work, I browsed through the testimonials I had posted on my website at the time. I thought about the clients I had *really* connected with and helped over the years.

It suddenly hit me like a post candy splurge sugar high: a whole bunch of people I helped were also health and wellness professionals. A physiotherapist, other dietitians, a massage therapist, a personal trainer, a nurse, a doctor… People who had enough healthy eating knowledge to know how to do this, but they got into trouble anyhow. Without realizing it, I had been helping them through their stuff with the tools I learned to help myself. And I was changing their lives for the better. Here is what they said:

"I want to thank Coach Irene who used her ninja-like coaching skills on me to help me figure out how I could get out of my own way."

"I love knowing that you're in my corner, and on those days where it feels more like the grind than something fun, I have this made-up voice in my head that is you I can hear cheering me on telling me that even though I don't want to, I will be happy I did. And then I do, and then I'm always happy I did."

"I'm pleased with what I have accomplished Irene, and I'm so grateful to you for having coached me along the way. I've come out of the experience forever changed and a happier person for it."

I got curious about the patterns in these clients (and myself). You might think that being a nutrition expert would make it less likely for you to land yourself in trouble with eating and make it easier for you to get out of it if you do, right? Me too. Yet, it didn't seem to work that way. I saw these common struggles show themselves in different ways over and over again:

Inconveniences of Being Human

Your body doesn't know you've studied to fill your brain with amazing nutrition knowledge. Your nutrition expert body still wants and needs the same basic stuff as the body that belongs to a human who has not studied nutrition. It still plays by the same psychological and physiological rules. When you are an expert at something, it is easy to believe that you are somehow immune from suffering the same fate as the clients you serve. This belief can get you into trouble when it causes you to place super human expectations on yourself and obscure you from seeing the reality of the situation you're in. No matter how educated and skilled you are at your craft, you can't hack everything about being human. You have to learn strategies to deal, just like everybody else does. As Dr. E so eloquently put it, you are susceptible to the same "inconveniences of being human" as everyone else – even with regard to your eating – welcome to the club.

Misaligned Expectations, Ownership, and Action

Three specific challenges or misalignments show up again and again. I focused on resetting these for myself and my clients, other things seemed to flow more easily:

1. Shrink the distance between where you are now and where you think you should be. (Expectations)

2. Move from using external drivers and rules to internal values and principles to guide your eating choices. (Ownership)
3. Close the gap between knowing and doing. (Action)

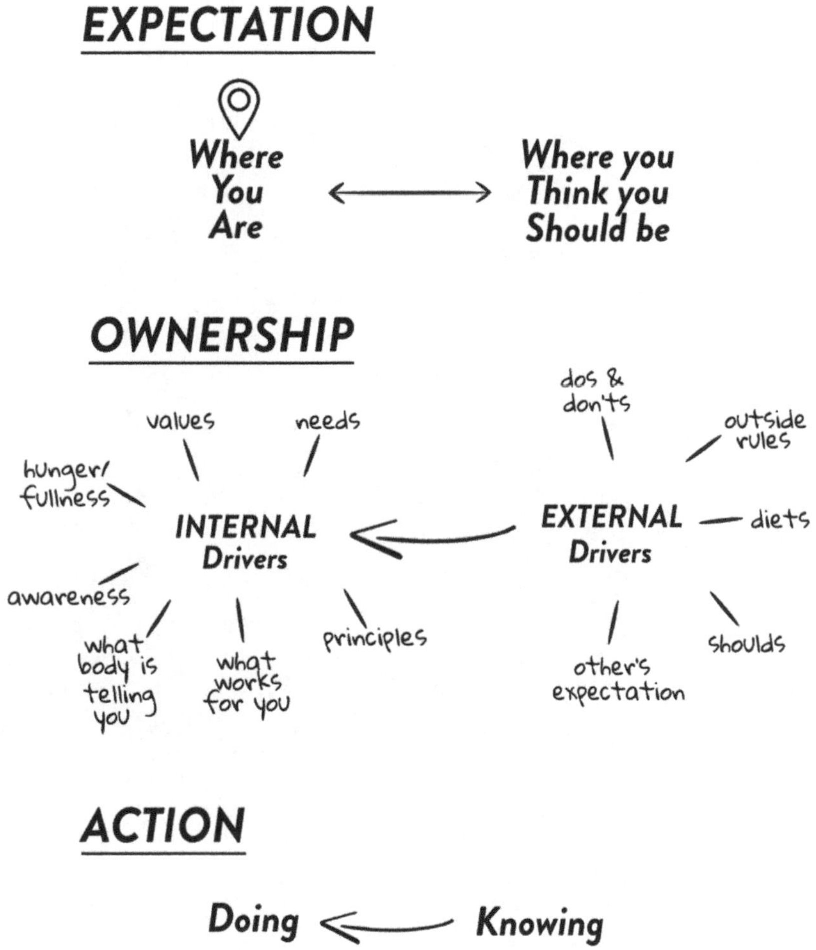

Another thing about being human, is to want to help people. I have that one. I've consumed countless courses and workshops and books and podcasts. I've worked with a number of brilliant coaches and put in years of personal and professional growth focused on figuring this out. Now, I want to use what I've learned to help you figure it out. That's exactly what I'm here to do in *Eat Like You Teach*.

Chapter 3:

Follow Instructions - An Owner's Manual Made by You for You

"Taking care of yourself doesn't mean me first, it means me too."

- L.R. Knost

You will be tuning in, experimenting, evaluating, trying things on, and learning a whole lot about yourself and what works best for your body and your life. By following the system in this book and capturing your key learnings as you go, you will create an Owner's Manual for yourself. A collection of operating or handling instructions unique to you that you can refer to and build out over time as you grow and change.

Think for a minute about the Owner's Manual for your blender. You might find basic operating instructions, a quick start guide, a maintenance manual, warnings and safety precautions, and probably a troubleshooting guide of some sort. The whole purpose of the Owner's Manual is to give you handling instructions for your blender so you can keep it functioning well. Follow the instructions and you have the best chance of it working beautifully. Ignore the instructions, skip the maintenance, and don't heed the safety precautions, and it should be no surprise that it won't perform optimally or at all as you expect. It will probably breakdown sooner than the lifespan it was designed to have. If you read the Manual for another blender (or a version of that same blender from five years ago) and try to apply those instructions to the blender in front of you, that likely won't work well either. Makes sense, right?

Let's apply the same concepts to *your* Owner's Manual. Basic operating instructions will give you clear steps to follow each day to make you a well-functioning human. These might be daily routines or setting your environment up best to serve you. You may have warnings and safety precautions for the places you know you are most likely to get into trouble. These might look like personal guidelines or guardrails or unique dos and don'ts that you've learned from experimenting. Perhaps you have quick start guidelines to get you going again when you've fallen off track or you're stuck in the grind. A maintenance manual will include essential self-care practices that keep you functioning at your best. You'd have a troubleshooting guide to turn to when you don't know *what* is going on but you know *something* is off.

The objective of writing your Owner's Manual is to give you handling instructions to be consistent and persistent at taking actions that are best for your body and your life. Just like it's essential to use the right Manual for the blender that is in front of you, you want to be using the right Manual for *you*. Not the Manual for your neighbor, or your colleague at work who lost thirty pounds, or some Instagram guru, or your mother, or the twenty-year-old version of you (unless you *are* twenty, of course). It's therefore essential as you go through this process of creating your Manual, that you think about creating it as honestly as you can in the context of your current life as it is, right now.

In order to truly do that, you'll be asked to be open to seeing things about yourself that you may have missed before. To be open to trying new things and evaluating what really works for you (not what you really want to work for you) and what doesn't. It ain't going to be comfy. It can't be. I'll be here with you along the way. If you get stuck reach out to me.

This process asks you to push through fears and make mistakes. It asks you to challenge stories and beliefs you have about yourself and what is right for you. Some of these narratives will have been with you for a long time. You will learn tools to tap into patience and compassion to help you along the way. This process requires you to fall down, so you can know what trips you up, and then get back up so you know how to do that too.

Setbacks and challenges are expected, normal, and even necessary. That doesn't make them easy, but it can help you re-frame them to be useful instead of discouraging. You will have exhilarating wins and ah-ha moments, and get to know the bravery it takes to face challenges head-on and the thrill of figuring it out. You learn a lot about yourself when you experience both of these. Experiencing what *doesn't* work is an essential step on your journey to find what *does*.

Once you discover those things that work for you, it's time to put them into action. Tune into what helps you to be more consistent and persistent and do more of that. Look at what gets in the way of being consistent and persistent and clear those things out. You learn to automate as many tasks as you can and set your environment up to support that.

As you work through the steps in this book, how you record your Manual is totally up to you. But writing it *somewhere* is essential. Remember that inconvenience of being human thing? Yeah that. If you don't record what you do here, you will forget it. The *act* of recording in and of itself is also a key part of the process. Recording allows you the opportunity to reflect and see patterns emerge that you may otherwise miss. A journal, notebook, or binder are the most common ways my clients keep their Owner's Manual (I use a notebook). Use an electronic method if you prefer (like Word, Pages, or Evernote) or you can even get creative and scrapbook it if that's your style. Don't let *how* your record become a big make-work project but do pick *something* that will allow you to capture data and learnings as you go.

Consider it a living document; add to and revise it as your body and your life change and as you learn and discover new things about yourself. You will have one central place to capture the cyclical patterns around when the trouble spots come up for you. It could be seasonal: it could be related to extra busy time at work or for family things or maybe even holidays that affect you in a certain way.

Paying attention to, reflecting on, and recording will help you see patterns and better prepare and navigate when the same or similar challenges come up in the future. If you approach difficult times as an opportunity to build out your Owner's Manual, it can be a powerful re-frame where you focus on the thrill of growth and discovery that comes on the other side of the hard stuff.

The chapters in *Eat Like You Teach* are organized into four main sections. They're not steps that need to be followed in any particular order but principles and a framework to navigate from. The first time you read through this book, it will be easiest to follow if you read in the order it is presented. After that, the headings used throughout allow you to skim along the surface and find the section that is most pertinent to you in the moment. Pop in and out of the book for reference as needed.

Part I: Reality

I share with you the piece of my story that got me here, the solution I discovered along the way and how I am going to teach you my system to find your own way through this.

Chapter 2: Be Human - Like You Have a Choice

Chapter 3: Follow Instructions - An Owner's Manual Made by You for You

Part II: Reboot

This is the system and principles that you will use in creating your Owner's Manual.

Chapter 4: Start Here - Make Your Expectations Work for You

Chapter 5: Get Curious - Awareness, Curiosity and Compassion

Chapter 6: Try Stuff - Experiment and Evaluate

Part III: Reset

You will learn how to apply the principles from Part II to figure out what works best for your body and your life and build that into your Owner's Manual.

Chapter 7: Eat Better - Five Steps to Reset Your Eating

Chapter 8: Boost Energy - Move and Sleep Like Your Life Depends On It

Chapter 9: Cultivate Environment - Create an Operating Space that Supports You

Part IV: Reclaim

In this section you will learn tools and strategies to put the handling instructions in your Owner's Manual into action.

Chapter 10: Take Action - Turn Knowing into Doing

Chapter 11: Steer Dynamically - Navigate Common Obstacles

Chapter 12: Own It - You Got This

I'm excited to bring you the system and principles that helped me through when I needed a reset. They continue to be the principles and systems I live by today.

By learning the process, you will have powerful tools that can serve you into the future because when your life and your body change, it will be time to update your Manual and you will know exactly how to do that.

Part II:

Reboot

Chapter 4:

Start Here – Make Your Expectations Work for You

"1.4 A: Don't get hung up on your views of how things 'should' be because you will miss out on learning how they really are."
– Ray Dalio, Principles

Let's start at the beginning. The best place to begin is where you are now. It's the *only* place to begin, really. You can't start where you used to be or where you wish you were, but sometimes your mind likes to make you think you can. Stepping into the reality of "*what is*" is an essential principle for building an Owner's Manual that you can rely on. If you build your Owner's Manual based on where you were at a previous time in your life or where you think you should or want to be, you'll be building the wrong manual. It will be for somebody else's life or the wrong version of your life. Certainly, use past experiences to inform what you choose to do now; you'd be missing out on learning from them if you didn't. At the same time, expectations that what worked then *should* work now can get you into trouble. Expectations in general can get you into trouble, and that's why I'll give you tools to get them working for you instead of against you in this chapter.

Start Where You Are

You want the most current version of your Owner's Manual, the one that takes into account your body and your life right now. It's therefore essential that you build it in the context of the realities you encounter in your life right now. As it is, not as you wish it were or as you think it should be – what it *is*.

Show up with the intention of wanting to know the truth about your reality (as difficult as that may be sometimes). It doesn't do you any good to hide from the truth about your life. Correct that: it doesn't do you any good to hide from the truth about your life if you want to change it. Any good outcome is rooted in an accurate understanding of reality. Start from here, the place you *actually* live, now. Here are some principles for starting where you are:

Practice a beginner's mindset

Life as you know it right now is not exactly as it was a year ago or a day ago or even a moment ago (if you want to get super technical and a little woo-woo). It's continually evolving and changing, and this is where those who approach with a beginner's mindset come out on top. Beginner's mindset means you approach any situation with the underlying belief that you have something to learn. It's much easier to learn if you believe there is something to learn.

This is especially true in the "expert" space, where it's easy to feel a pull to be the person who has all the answers especially in your area of expertise. Do you know someone who responds to everything with a version of "I already knew that?" Right. Don't be that guy. The more of a master you truly become, the more you realize how little you know and just how much there is still to learn. Open yourself to the idea that, although it used to be X way, it is totally possible that Y is the way is it now. Or that you believe *A* to be true but can entertain the possibility that *B* (or something else you have yet to discover) may also be true. And if that is the case, you want to know.

Writer and artist Brian Andreas says, "It doesn't help to listen carefully if you're only going to listen for stuff you already know." With each new learning, you get to begin again with a new perspective. Be open to see the next thing you don't yet know, and it will find you more easily.

Embrace a growth mindset

If beginner's mindset is that you believe you have *something to learn*, growth mindset is when you believe you *can learn*. The opposite of growth mindset is fixed mindset. Fixed mindset says you're born smart (or not). You know what you know (or not). You can't teach an old dog new tricks. That's a pretty difficult (almost impossible) place to change and grow from. Growth aside, it creates loads of unnecessary struggle, feelings of failure, and hopelessness in life to go around believing that you can't grow.

In a growth mindset, you believe that even the most basic, seemingly innate abilities can be developed and expanded through specific and deliberate practice. This fosters a desire for, and love of, learning and practice. The belief that you can learn and grow through something difficult can fuel determination and resilience and allow you to continue to move forward even at times it seems like everything is pushing you not to. Combine this with a belief that experiences in life, no matter how light or dark, are an opportunity to learn something, and you are set to get through anything.

Check Your Expectations

Expectations matter (a lot). They can set you on a path to tremendous growth, or they can hold you in a place of suffering. The beauty and the burden of this is that you alone are in control of *your* expectations. You get to choose to hold expectations that help you or hurt you, but you can only make a choice if you're aware of them. When you hear words like these from yourself or others, know that expectations are lurking, and use them as a trigger to tune in: *must, have to, need to, supposed to, had better, should*. You may discover you are *should-ing* on yourself all day long.

Why does that matter? Shoulds have a big impact on how successful you feel. If every little success is crowded out by all the *shoulds* that were not looked after, you can see it becomes easy to feel like you never get to enjoy any successes at all. "I did have a great breakfast today, but I shouldn't have stopped for a latte on my way to work, and I've got to get better a drinking more water, and I was supposed to pack my lunch for today, but I didn't." Success breeds success, but not a lot of breeding will happen in the dark land of *shoulds*.

If you discover you are running around with superhuman expectations in every area of life – your eating, movement, sleep, relationships, work – you are not alone. As you tune in, you will see how some expectations serve you and some don't. As much as you would love them to, superhuman expectations don't necessarily make things go faster. They may actually get in the way of progress.

ex·pec·ta·tion
/ˌekspekˈtāSH(ə)n/
noun
a strong belief that something will happen or be the case in the future.
a belief that someone will or should achieve something.

So, what do you do? You practice checking in with your expectations as you go about building your Owner's Manual (and the rest of your life). Ask yourself questions like, "What are my expectations right now? Do I believe this expectation belongs to me or someone else? What is influencing what I expect? Does it make sense? Does this expectation serve me? Does it serve somebody else?" It demands frequent tuning in and adjusting course. Expectations are sneaky little things.

I had no idea just how much my expectations were impacting my life until I started tuning in. I had humongous, unrealistic (and crushing) expectations weighing me down in some places. I had humongous, inspiring (and helpful) expectations lifting me up in other places. Once I started to unpack them, I soon realized some belonged to me and a bunch belonged to others (family, work, society at large). Some were fairly new, and some had been with me a long (*long*) time. As a dietitian, the expectations I had about what my own eating *should* look like needed a significant reset. I remember realizing on a call with Coach Pam that I basically had a deep gnawing expectation that I should be laying out a dinner spread like Martha Stewart each night in order to be a successful Dietitian Mother. Right. That was helpful. There is a lot of room between a Martha Stewart-worthy spread and toaster oven English muffin pizzas.

Think for a minute about what you expect from yourself in terms of eating. And then think about what you expect from your clients or your colleagues or any other human that is not you. Notice anything? Do you believe your expectations are helping you, moving you further ahead? Is there room to close the gap a little there – between where you are and where you think you should be?

Here are few expectations that will serve you *well* in the process of creating your Owner's Manual (and perhaps in the process of living in general):

Expect it to be difficult, uncomfortable, and to downright suck at times

Bring to mind something you've done that was difficult that you *knew* would be difficult. Perhaps you ran a race or signed up for a super intense workout at the gym. Or you started a new job or project that you knew would test your limits. Or you delivered a baby (that's an easy pick if you have that one on your resume). Are you with me here?

Now think about something you've done that was difficult, and you thought it *wouldn't be.* Maybe you even thought it would be easy, and it ended up totally not being easy. How did you show up differently for the first difficult thing compared to the second? Both are difficult, but the expectations around each were different. How do you show up differently when you *expect* something to suck? When you sign on for it *knowing* it will suck?

I can hear you saying, "Okay, Irene, but some difficulties are more difficult than other difficulties." And I get that; you're right. Right now, where you are and the struggles you're having are difficult, no question. Yet, suppose for a minute you believed you are exactly where you are meant to be. What if life is *supposed* to go like this? Exactly like this. If you changed the thought in your head about this hard thing from "This sucks, and it shouldn't" to "This sucks, and it should," how would you show up differently?

You know this, but I'm going to say it anyhow. Change requires discomfort. You cannot grow from a place of comfort. If you want change – which I know you do because you're here – you can fight the discomfort, or you can expect that it is part of the process, lean in, and get it over with. You get to narrow that gap between how it is and how you think it *should* be by shifting your expectations. If you want to.

Expect to have blind spots

You have blind spots even though you don't like to think you do. There are things about yourself that you can't see, areas where your way of thinking prevents you from a complete and accurate view of reality, no matter how hard you try. It's not special to you; blind spots are a human thing. Expecting that you can't see it all and you can't appreciate what you can't see creates room to be open to observations and feedback from others in a new way. Feedback and *outside eyes* stop being something to fear and become something worth seeking out (if you really want to see the truth, that is).

This video called "It's Not About the Nail" puts this concept on display in a fantastic (and hilarious) way https://www.youtube.com/watch?v=-4EDhdAHrOg. Expect to have blind spots. Hold space for the idea that you may not see something that is plainly obvious to someone else. Not all feedback has the same weight or is deserving of your time, but seeking to understand what people in your life who truly have your best intentions at heart observe may save you from unnecessary struggle and pain and may strengthen pieces of your Owner's Manual.

Expect to have control of *your* actions

It is easy to have faulty expectations around control. You live in a world that feeds the idea that you can and should take control of every aspect your life. The trouble is that can cause you to spend your precious time and energy in places that you cannot possibly, and will never, have control over.

Getting clear on your expectations around control will serve you well because you can choose to place your energy where it really *can* make a difference in your life. You can eliminate a large amount of unnecessary struggle that comes with trying to control things that are not yours to control. Here is an exercise to help you sort out which things to focus your energy the most.

Spheres of Control

On a blank piece of paper, draw three circles as follows:

1. A large circle filling most of the page. Label it "No control"
2. Inside that circle, draw a smaller circle. Label it "Some control."
3. Inside the second circle, draw a third smaller circle. Label it "Total control"

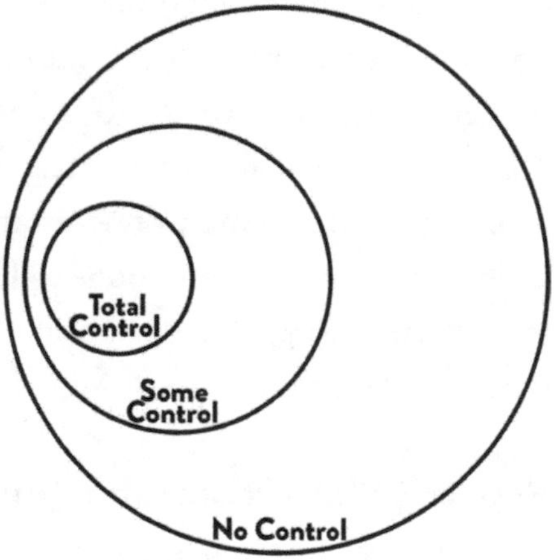

Write in each circle, things in your life that fit each category. Things like the weather and traffic and what others think or say to you – many of the things that can cause you stress or suck your energy, are in the "No control" circle. Your thoughts, your schedule, everyday routines, may fall in the "Some Control" circle. Few things may fall in the total control circle but a key one does fall there – your actions. Humm…I wonder would happen if you channelled all of your "control" energy *there*?

Expect others' expectations to masquerade as your own

You will feel the pull of the expectations of others (or social norms of the day). You already have your hands full shuffling and sorting the expectations you create for yourself; let them do the same with their own. When you identify an expectation, see if you can instantly decide if it really belongs with you. The Owner's Manual process can help you move from using external drivers and rules to internal values and guidelines for your eating choices – if you let it. Clearing the expectations of others out of your path can help smooth the way.

Expect the *expected* unexpected

Surprise! You overate again at Thanksgiving dinner. Surprise! When you went into the break room on treat day, you ate two donuts and a brownie. Surprise! You're eating every sugary carb you can get your hands on three days before your period starts. The realities you encounter are repetitive. Some repeat more frequently than others, but for the most part, there is more predictability in the unexpected than your brain allows you to believe there is. On one hand, you know these unexpected things are getting in the way of your goals. On the other hand, calling them unexpected means you get to be a victim to them and don't have to expect yourself to do anything about them. It feels icky to acknowledge that, but as much as this hinders you, it also serves you, right? It means you cannot be held accountable to your actions. It is a kind way to give yourself an easy out – "I didn't know!" "I was caught off guard."

As you get curious in your Owner's Manual process, get curious about the patterns in these unexpected realities of your life. Don't allow yourself to be surprised and be victim to things that are not really a surprise at all. Get these things in your Owner's Manual. Record how often they tend to happen. Look at how you've handled that (or other things like that) in the past and what worked and what didn't. Practice pausing and making your action a choice, and see what happens. There is power in owning your choice even if that choice is to eat three donuts on treat day. So the next time it happens, instead of being all, "Oh my gosh! You won't believe what happened!" be all, "There's this thing again. I got this. I choose X this time."

Expect that part of being human is dealing with B.S.

From a young age, you are led to believe that a good happy life is a life mostly free from trouble and strife, that feeling blissfully happy, almost all the time, is the destination to strive for. You can imagine yourself running, arms outstretched, through a field of flowers. This is not about bursting bubbles or being pessimistic (I might be one of the most optimistic people on the planet). It's about giving you every opportunity to actually live the real version of your happiest life. The version that includes moving through joy and bliss and dark and difficult, the version that includes happiness despite the ridiculous number of horrible things that happen in your life and everyone else's all the time, from now until you die.

As my mentor Angela Lauria so eloquently put it, "And that's never ever going to change. No day in the future when it's changing. There's no amount of money, there's no new husband, there's no computer gadget. Fifty percent of being human is dealing with B.S. News flash."

An expectation of perpetual bliss creates additional, unnecessary struggle in a world that gives us enough. It gets in the way of being free to learn how to embrace and celebrate your normal life in all its mess and glory. Think about building your Owner's Manual in the context of your real life, one that includes regular B.S. and stuff going sideways. If you build your Manual based on your *perfect* day – when all the stars align, the kids and dog and partner are happy, you hit all the green lights on the way to the office – you won't be able to rely on it most of the time.

Expect trade-offs and choose yours

Getting back in alignment is a lot about trade-offs. Not trade-offs that others force you to make, trade-offs you *get* to make based on what matters most to you. Everything comes at the cost of something else: cost of time, opportunity cost because doing one thing means you are not doing something else. When you expect trade-offs, you give yourself the opportunity to be deliberate about choosing the trade-off you want to make. You get to choose to spend your energy and time in the places that matter most to you.

When you allow yourself to expect to do all the things, you rob yourself of making that choice. When it comes to your health and fitness and nutrition, there are trade-offs just like everywhere else. Precision Nutrition created a fantastic infographic that shows different levels of leanness for Men and Women and gives guidelines about what it takes to get there. It's titled *The Cost of Getting Lean.* Take a look:

https://www.precisionnutrition.com/cost-of-getting-lean-infographic

Based on this model, what would you have to do *more* of and what would you have to do *less* of based on where you want to be? It may be a sobering look at how your expectations align with the rest of your life. How much do you *really* want to focus on eating a specific way, and optimizing sleep and exercise as part of your life? What would you have to give up or trade-off in order to do that? Take a look and see where you are. There is no right or wrong answer; that's the whole point. Take a look at the graphic, think about what level of fitness and leanness you want, and see if the steps needed to get there are in alignment with the other things that matter in your life right now.

My goal in this book is to help you clear the path to health and nutrition alignment in your life. I can give you some clear and simple steps, but I can't make them all easy even if I wanted to. You can change how your journey feels by practicing seeing and stepping into your reality and checking if the expectations you hold for yourself are helping you or hurting you. Build your Owner's Manual based on the real life you are living now. Adjust your *expectations* to shrink the gap and tension between where you are and where you think you should be. Create a greater level of *ownership* and *alignment* by moving from external drivers and rules to internal values and guidelines around food and eating. Take *action,* and close that gap between what you know and what you do.

Chapter 5:

Get Curious - Awareness, Curiosity, and Compassion

"To wonder is to begin to understand."
- José Ortega y Gasset

After you've stepped into your reality and expectations, it's time to pause and take a look around. Take stock of what life looks like for you. That look can bring you all kinds of valuable information that is essential for building your Owner's Manual. Awareness and curiosity are key ingredients to make that happen. Self-compassion allows you to look with kindness versus judgment and therefore makes it more likely that you will look often and honestly. Honing these skills won't happen all on its own; you've got to get deliberate about it. The good news is:

- No matter where you are starting from, these skills can be built.
- Big grand gestures are not needed. Small actions (whenever you can make them) make a difference.
- It's worth every ounce of effort you give it.

Set Up Triggers To Practice

Building a new skill of any kind requires that you do the behavior again and again and again – practice. Often the practice itself is not difficult but *remembering* to do it can be. That makes strategies and systems that prompt you to practice super valuable. Creating triggers to practice is a tool that has been instrumental in successful change for both my clients and me.

By connecting your desired new practice with an event or action that already happens as part of your normal day, you create a trigger for the new action. The key is to pick a trigger that is specific and immediately actionable. Awareness, curiosity, and compassion can be practiced anywhere, anytime and need only take an instant, so there are endless opportunities to practice. Win!

James Clear identifies five types of habit cues (or triggers): time, location, preceding event, emotional state, and other people (more here: https://jamesclear.com/habit-triggers). This may sound complicated, but it doesn't have to be. You can do a fast version of this right now. Grab a paper, and draw a line down the middle, making two columns. In the first column, write a list of things that automatically happen already in your day (e.g. red light, your phone pings); in the other column, write a list of things that you already do every day consistently (e.g. you brush your teeth, you go to the bathroom, you make a cup of tea, you eat meals). Look at your list, and pick one thing that you could use at trigger for awareness. One of my first ones was standing up or sitting down from my desk. Standing or sitting is the trigger to tune in and ask myself, "What is going on for me right now?" I ask with curiosity and bring in self-compassion if what I see stirs up the mean girl in me.

BJ Fogg, the creator of Tiny Habits, has a fantastic little formula to help build habits and group actions together. It goes like this, "1. After I ____ … 2. Then I'll ____." Simple but super effective, right?

Take that one for a test drive. If you want more of this from BJ Fogg, check out his Tedx talk: https://youtu.be/AdKUJxjn-R8.

Awareness

This chapter comes before the one about experimenting for a reason. At first, practice awareness all on its own without any requirement to do anything at all about what you learn or see. There's no pressure or requirement to change anything or make a different choice based on what you observe. Just observe. Get curious about it. And be nice (compassionate) to yourself about it. What helps you to be more aware? What gets in the way? Add that to your Owner's Manual and practice. Keep the pressure of *shoulds* and *change* off the table all together. There is plenty of time for that.

a•ware•ness
/əˈwernəs/
noun
knowledge or perception of a situation or fact.

Imagine yourself standing outside on a day with a slight breeze. You've been asked which way the wind is blowing. You pause for a minute and can't quite tell. You could make a guess and get it over with, but you are pretty sure you will have missed something if you do. So you wet a finger and place it up in the air and… tune in and… wait.

That is the quality of awareness you're looking for. Pause and see what comes. Feel the pull to snap to an answer and wait anyhow. Here are ways to practice and hone your awareness skills. Give them a try and add the ones that work for you to your Owner's Manual:

Pause

I've already mentioned taking a pause a number of times. That's because this is one of the most powerful little tools you can arm yourself with. There is tremendous power in the pause. Pause. Pause before you eat. Pause before you speak. Pause before you act in that way you want to change. In that little moment of pause, you disrupt a well-worn default pathway in your brain and create room to bring the power of choice into the equation. You can feel the pull towards a behavior, but you don't have to go there. It's so simple, right? Yet, it's so not easy. "Excruciatingly difficult" fits a little better at times. But man, there is so much power in the pause. Set up triggers to pause. Practice this guy anywhere and everywhere, and before you know it – pause – it will become your default.

Notice And Name

When you notice something about yourself – a feeling, an emotion, a thought – practice naming it. "What's going on for me right now?" A feelings wheel can be helpful when you can't seem to find words (which is normal, by the way, especially when you are new to this practice).

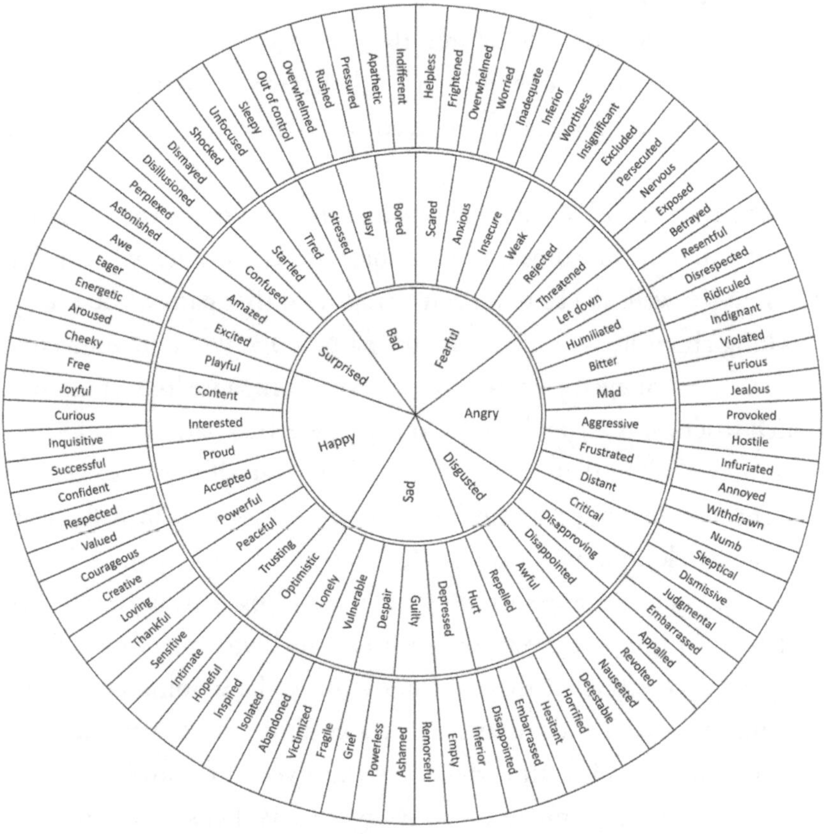

Printed with permission from Geoffrey Roberts

If a name doesn't seem to fit, you may also try describing what it is "like" instead. "It's like this knot in my stomach" or "It's like I want to scream but can't". The power of this practice is less about getting it right and more about the power of putting words to your feelings or emotions, any words. And they don't have to make sense to anyone, not even you (How's that for a zero-pressure game?).

Practice your notice and name all on its own without the pull to have to make a change or do something about it.

See The Path

If imagery works well for you, this strategy may work too. When you turn up your awareness about a behavior or thought pattern, imagine it's like standing at the head of a well-worn path in a field of tall grass.

The path (your default or habitual behavior) is the easy choice – even if you don't like or want that choice. It's right there, clear as day. You know it well. For so long, you've followed that path without even thinking about it. When you see this path, when you find yourself at the head of it or even partway down it, you can pause long enough to notice where you are and say, "I know where this path leads. I know how this ends." In that moment, you allow yourself a choice. Choose to continue on the path you know or choose to step into the long grass and trek out a new path. At first, just notice the path.

Tune your awareness to the sequence of how you have travelled that path in the past, how you get to it, and where it leads, all the familiar pieces about it that you know so well. At some point, you may make the difficult and uncomfortable choice to step off the path. It is unfamiliar and unclear right now, and you don't know where it leads, but you may choose to do it anyway. Perhaps that is because you now know the discomfort or pain following the old path creates for you. Perhaps that discomfort is now greater than the fear of the unknown new path, and you are willing to take a chance. There is no rule that says because you choose the new path *this time* that you have to choose it *next time*. Every time, it's your choice to make. Suppose you wanted to take a different path one of these times; what might that look like? How might you start?

With enough passes along a new path, the old one will begin to grow over and fade, and the new one will become clearer. It takes time and consistency, and the first many passes require you to deliberately take the harder road. The first essential step is seeing the worn path so you can open yourself to the possibility that you may want to go a different way. Start there and see what happens.

A Slow Glass Of Water

This practice is specifically about finetuning (or waking up) your internal physical awareness. Being an athlete most of my life, I believed I was someone who was pretty physically aware overall. When I was asked to tune into my hunger and fullness cues during my year as a nutrition client, it was crickets. My first thoughts were, "What?! *Really?* How can I be so terrible at this?! And how can I not *know* I am so terrible at this?!" As I widened my scope, I realized just how fantastic I was at tuning *out* or *distracting* myself from *all kinds* of internal messages (and feelings – *gulp*). I had years (maybe a lifetime) of practice burying them with busy tasks, phone checking, social media scrolling, or eating. I was a master. Well, it was time to become a master at tuning *in*.

This simple practice that I continue today was a game changer. I put a glass of water on my bedside table before I turn in each night and drink it first thing in the morning. I don't just guzzle it down; I pause and drink it mindfully. I feel the glass on my lips (temperature, texture) and where the first splash of water hits my mouth and the sensation as it travels down into my stomach. Cold water heightens all these sensations, so go ahead and use an insulated container if you like (Bonus: it may save you from dumping open glasses of water all over the pile of self-help books stacked on your night table).

What I love about this practice is that you get to change for yourself in three key ways with one glass of water: 1) You practice becoming aware of internal sensations, feelings inside your body, as you follow the water down (Note: you may not be able to feel those internal sensations at all at first. Carry on; it will come. Trust me on this.), 2) You practice being comfortable pausing and doing nothing but paying attention (Yes, this can be super uncomfortable at first.), 3) You can set the intention with that one drink at the beginning of the day to practice being more aware and present throughout the day.

Go *All In* On The Thing You Are Doing

This is the language that works to get me present with the task I am working on. For instance, right now I am *all in* on writing. My phone is off. My email and desktop notifications are off. My manuscript document is the only one I have open. I can easily discard thoughts that arise that are not about my writing by reminding myself, "I'm all in on *this* right now." When I started on this journey and would ask myself to be present or mindful, my brain would find workarounds or loopholes to make it okay for me to be working on or thinking about many things at once. With *all in,* I find I can't do that. I can't be *all in* on more than one thing at a time because that would mean I'm *not* all in. See how that works? Another way to frame this is single-tasking. You focus on one thing at a time, and if you are focusing on more than one, you are not single-tasking. My daughter walked in to ask me something just now; I stopped writing and went *all in* on listening to and having a conversation with her. I turned in my chair, looked at her, and we had our conversation. Now, I'm back here, all in on writing. This felt like such a concrete, manageable starting point for me. Even though I'm further along the path with my awareness and ability to be present than I was a few years ago, this is still my best way to get there. Try this one and see how it works for you and play around with what words are a solid cue to get and keep your present.

Meditation Practice

I avoided meditation practice in any real way for the longest time. I found all kinds of reasons and excuses as to why I couldn't or didn't need to do it. Old Irene was someone who was constantly go, go, go. Driving and striving. I was much more comfortable feeling like I was doing something purposeful. When I went for a walk, it felt better if it had a destination or was labeled in my head as deliberate exercise. When I would watch a movie, it felt right to also have my laptop beside me with some work to do or a basket of laundry to fold while I watched. I know now that all the manufactured busyness came from two places (perhaps you can relate):

1. I felt like I was of value and worth in the world if I was doing something that could be labeled as productive (up for debate how productive it all actually was).
2. Sitting alone, quiet with myself, with nothing to do seemed excruciating (that's a hard reality to face).

The very first habit I took on when I started working with Coach Pam was meditation.

I found an app called Headspace (https://www.headspace.com/). It was approachable and simple, complete with cute little cartoons and a pleasant dude with a great British accent to talk me through things. It is a fantastic tool to kickstart a new meditation practice for someone who is on the fence about a meditation practice in the first place.

I started with their guided process of ten minutes per day. What I really liked was being talked through things so even though I was not doing anything, I was doing something because I had instructions to follow along the way. It was helpful to think about it like exercise for my mind (which is actually not inaccurate at all). I meditated for forty-one days straight (was pretty proud of that) and over the rest of my coaching year with Pam meditated over 250 days (big win).

I noticed a shift in my focus and sense of inner calm or groundedness after the first month. It made tuning in and noticing things in my life less difficult with some of the noise in my head removed. My meditation practice became inconsistent for about six months. I allowed other things to take priority, and I stopped making time for even that ten minutes. Your Owner's Manual is going to reduce your risk of making the same mistake because if something works for you, if it makes a positive difference in your life, you will put it in your Owner's Manual and be reminded of that when you check in with your Manual.

I rebooted my meditation practice when a friend introduced me to Sam Harris's work and his meditation app called Waking Up (https://wakingup.com/). His approach and deeper dive into consciousness totally hit the mark for me, and a ten-minute, focused meditation is a non-negotiable part of my day. What has been surprisingly powerful is the idea that meditation does not require a build-up or ritual to begin (e.g. sit a specific way, take breaths for x amount of time, visualize, or state your intent etc.). There certainly is a place for practice like that, but it is freeing to know you can still exercise your brain and advance your meditation practice without that. You can make great progress with a practice of "dropping into consciousness" in an instant, anytime, anywhere. I apply that in moments in my day all over the place now (not when I'm driving). It has been an extremely helpful way to train my awareness.

When you read all the hype about how meditation practice can change your life, take notice. You don't have to shave your head and hang out in robes while sitting cross-legged on the floor to get the benefit. It's more about a chance to practice tuning in, like a workout session to build your awareness muscle. Awareness is a non-negotiable principle in growth and change. So if you have an interest in some growth and change stuff (which I'm guessing you do because you're here), meditation isn't a waste of time; it's a productive and useful practice (okay, still working on this one).

Curiosity

Awareness and curiosity are similar but not the same. While awareness is the desire to have knowledge or perception of something, to *see* it, curiosity is the desire to know or learn something. It's a dynamic duo, first seeing and then learning from whatever it is you are focusing on. Helpful phrases so spark curiosity include: "I wonder…" "Do I believe…?" "Isn't that curious?" "Is it possible that…?"

cu·ri·os·i·ty
/ˌkyo͝orēˈäsədē/
noun
a strong desire to know or learn something.

What to get curious about:

Get Curious About Patterns

Humans are creatures of habit, and although things in your day may seem random and unexpected – especially now when you are struggling with your eating – you may be surprised that there are still many patterns to be found: realities you encounter over and over again, patterns in your thoughts, feelings, emotions, and behaviors, broad sweeping patterns over days or weeks or months or years, smaller more specific patterns connected to tasks and actions in your day. Get curious about patterns and see what you can uncover that you may not have been aware of before. Most of the actions that you would like to change don't happen in isolation. There is a series of events or steps that lead up to them. Seeing those patterns and stepping in to the reality of them gives you an entry point for making a change, if and when you'd like to do that. Ask yourself, "Suppose there was a pattern here for me; what might that be?"

If It's Hysterical, It's Historical

If it's hysterical, it's historical. Catchy little phrase that is a powerful reminder to get curious about what is going on when a big reaction comes. I practice using a big swell of emotion in me as a trigger to say to myself, "If it's hysterical, it's historical." (Sometimes it comes just *after* I've reacted... Oops! Cue the self-compassion). When you feel the pull to react in a way that is logically disproportionate to the actual event you've just experienced, there is a good chance the reaction is stemming from somewhere else (your childhood? a past relationships or similar incident?). Getting curious can uncover all kinds of interesting things about yourself and create a space to pause and decide if you would like to choose a different way, if you would like to be a different person in response to that same trigger. Perhaps there is a story you tell yourself here that is due for a rewrite. Capture these things in your Owner's Manual. It may take some reflection, and perhaps some outside eyes, to get to the bottom of it, but it's worth it to get to a place where you can say, "Ah, here we go. Another one of these." And ride it out.

Explore How Your Problem Serves You

The places you feel stuck are often places you feel conflicted in some way, whether you realize it or not. What does this conflict look like? On one hand, you want X and, on the other hand, Y. PN taught me a tool called *Two Crazy Questions* (or *Speaking to the Monster*) to help tease out the conflict when it isn't totally clear. It goes like this:

First, what is *good* about *not* changing?

Second, what is *bad* about changing?

You see where this is going? The questions get at how this *problem* you want gone is also serving you in some way. This one can be really uncomfortable and stir up a whole bunch of shame. "What kind of messed up person am I that I *want* (insert undesirable thing)?" At the same time, it can also bring relief to see that it makes some sense and you are not actually messed up for keeping that habit around still (This is a great opportunity for self-compassion practice... We are headed there next). Ask yourself: Suppose I still have xx problem because I want to have it, because it is serving me in some way. What might that be? There is much to be learned in the stuck places, so get curious here and keep track in your Owner's Manual.

What Else?

Asking, "What else?" is a simple but powerful little curiosity question. I use it all over the place and continue to be surprised just how often there *is* something else. "What else is here for me to learn?" and "What is this ___ (experience/feeling/relationship etc) asking me to look at in myself? What is this __ teaching me today?" Opening up to the idea that there may be something else there that is not yet in your consciousness is often all that is needed to help tease it out.

Self-Compassion

Dr. Rebecca Ray says, "What if, instead, you listened to the voice inside you that's kind and gentle?" This one is a toughie. Society, and perhaps your family, taught you that what you need is *tough love* and a mental butt-kicking from yourself to make it in the world. Handling yourself kindly and gently is seen as a weak and totally undesirable way to function in the world if you want to succeed. So it's not your fault that you walk around with a mean girl or tyrant coach in your head yelling down at you with a stream of "constructive" criticism all day long. You are trying to do what you were taught is best for you. Times like now when you are trying to solve a problem and struggling to get it together, you likely kick the "constructive" criticism into high gear.

Trouble is, that is the exact *opposite* of what you need to make change. Logically you *know* that. Professionally, you know that and have likely talked with your clients about not being so hard on themselves. Or perhaps, like me, you thought your self-compassion game was solid… until you realized it wasn't. Well good news, the stuff that comes up in your awareness and curiosity practice will give you *loads* of opportunity to practice self-compassion (silver lining). If you allow your inner critic to beat you up for the things you discover, it will make for tough days ahead. The truth is you deserve to have relief from suffering, too. You are the only person you are with 24/7. If another person spoke to you the way you speak to yourself, would you be spending that much time with them? Right. With all the awareness practice you're going to be doing, you will have lots of opportunities to have a good ol' heart to heart with that mean inner voice and learn to do it a little differently.

Self-compassion involves acting towards yourself, the same compassionate way you would towards others who are having a difficult time. Instead of just ignoring your pain with a "suck it up" mentality, you stop to tell yourself "this is really difficult right now," how can I comfort and care for myself in this moment? Self-compassion is a welcome side-kick to awareness. Curiosity can help you move into that non-judgmental place where self-compassion becomes a little less hard. Dr. Mark Hyman says that "[e]very cell in your body is listening to your thoughts." Unkind words and thoughts have an impact beyond just making you feel miserable. Honing your self-compassion game is well worth the effort.

About a year into the start of my big personal growth party, I attended a full day workshop with Kristin Neff, who is a pioneer in the field of self-compassion research. At her workshop, I finally *got* self-compassion for the first time in my adult life. Dr. Neff defines self-compassion as being made up of three components: kindness, common humanity, and mindfulness. Here's more on that:

Self-Kindness Versus Self-Judgment

- Treat yourself with care and understating rather than harsh judgment
- Actively sooth and comfort, support and protect yourself

Common Humanity Versus Isolation

- See your own experience as part of a larger human experience, not as isolating or abnormal
- Recognizing that life is imperfect (us too!)

Mindfulness Versus Over-Identification

- "Courageous present-ness"
- Allow yourself to "be" with painful feelings as they are (not resist or try to fix)
- Avoid the extremes of suppressing or running away with painful feelings

My three *big* takeaways from the self-compassion workshop were:

Practice Acceptance Of Your Perfectly Normal Imperfect Life

Recognize that an imperfect life is really the only kind of life there is. Catch the "this is not supposed to happen" feeling in you (see the section on expectations) and remember that things going "wrong" is part of the normal human condition. This *is* how it is supposed to be sometimes.

Your Inner Critic Can Show Up In Ways Other Than Negative-Self *Talk*

Much of the self-compassion stuff didn't connect for me because I could not locate the "mean girl" in my head. I have never been one to say, "Oh, you're such an idiot!" or "That was stupid!" or "You'll never get this right!" to myself. Which also means all the strategies to turn "mean girl" talk into use positive self-talk never resonated with me either.

We did an exercise where we tuned in to our inner critic, and I had an "ah-ha" moment when she asked us to consider what your inner critic *feels like*. What does your inner critic *feel* like? I discovered mine (note: awareness and curiosity at work) is a gnawing feeling deep in my body – not words in my head. She's the feelings that go with a seething glare, a head hung low in disappointment, a shameful finger-wagging, or a back deliberately and painfully turned in my direction. Not words.

It's worth spending some time figuring out what your inner-critic is like so you can line up the type of support you need from yourself to begin to 'speak' to him/her in a way that fits.

Touch Is A Powerful Means Of Providing Comfort And Self-Compassion

A system in your body called the *mammalian caregiver system* releases a hormone called oxytocin in response to touch. In a moment of distress, oxytocin helps you feel a sense of security, helps you feel calm, and physiologically brings down some of the unpleasant symptoms you can experience when you are feeling stressed or feeling bad. It all has to do with the amazing sensitivity of your skin and the power of touch. There is a way you may activate this system for yourself. It is essentially like giving yourself a hug. Okay so I get that sounds a little awkward, but bear with me here; it is not quite as bad as it sounds, and it is an amazing tool to have in your toolbox.

Here are two ways to practice self-compassion with touch (what Dr. Kneff refers to as "soothing touch"):

1. When experiencing a difficult emotion, scan your body for where you feel it most easily or the feeling expresses itself most strongly. Place a gentle hand over that part of your body while you say caring words to yourself, "this is really difficult right now."
2. Try a more general soothing gesture to look after yourself in moments of suffering. Experiment to find one that feels soothing for you – e.g. hand over heart, one hand on your cheek or cradling your face in hands, gently stroking your arms like a self-hug etc.

If this is a new practice for you, the caring words may be difficult to find. Here are two strategies to help you find the words.

Words to a dear friend

Imagine that a dear friend is having the same problem or difficult emotion that is causing you struggle or pain. What would you say to him or her? If there were a few words you would like your friend to carry with them when they go, what would you like those words to be? See if you can offer that same message to yourself.

Words from a loving grandparent

Imagine you have a loving grandparent to turn to with this struggle or pain. They receive you with open arms and offer loving words to help you though. What might those words be? What do you imagine they would say to you? Again, see how you might offer that same message to yourself.

Making a habit of being compassionate about what turns up in your awareness and curiosity practice allows you to build these essential skills at the same time and link them together – which really is an almost magical way of transforming your relationship with yourself.

Upping your awareness, curiosity, and self-compassion game will not only make your Owner's Manual more accurate and useful but can change your experience of what it's like to engage in personal growth for the better. Because why wouldn't you want to relieve pain and suffering when it is present? This is your life. Right now. You live it along the way. So you might as well practice living it with joy and kindness toward yourself, whenever you get that chance.

Chapter 6:

Try Stuff – Experiment and Evaluate

"All life is an experiment. The more experiments you make the better."

– Ralph Waldo Emerson

You are starting where you are. You have checked in and rebooted expectations so they serve both present and future you. By tuning in, getting curious, and being kind with what you see, you've learned some stuff about yourself and identified pieces you want in your Owner's Manual. So here you are at the experiment and evaluate part of the game. The fun part! You get to try stuff to figure out what works for you and what doesn't. Both successes and failures are equally necessary to get the job done.

Experiment

You won't know what will work until you try it. Since you're clever and know your nutrition stuff, it can be tempting to believe you can just think *harder* to figure this out. If that worked, you wouldn't be here. In fact, thinking harder can get in the way of finding the truth. So warm up your beginner's mindset and put on your scientist hat, and let's see what you can discover about yourself.

The focus of your experiments is to see what works for you. To create the content for your Owner's Manual so the reference you have for what to do, the handling instructions, are based on your body and your life right now. To know what *works* for you, you have to think about it in terms of what matters to you. Going to the gym six days per week may *work* for getting the body you want but that may *not work* in terms of spending time with your family. You no longer have to use somebody else's Manual or an outdated version of your own Manual. You can move away from external drivers and rules, in favor of internally guided values and principles. We'll be applying this process to your eating but it really applies to just about anything in your life, not just food.

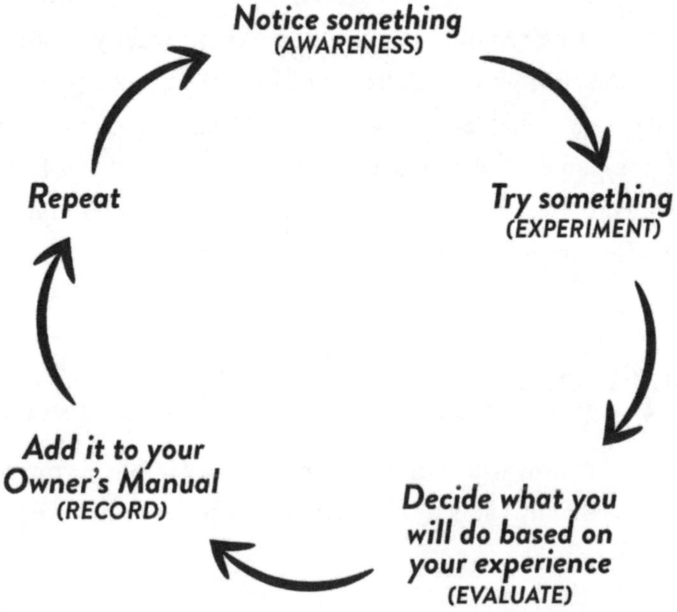

There are different methods or approaches for experimenting. You may find you like or lean towards one particular style or another. Or you may choose one type in one case and something else the next time. What's most important is taking *action* and doing what works best for *you* (you've heard that before, huh?).

Principles and strategies for experimentation:

Discomfort Is The Birthplace Of Growth

Discomfort is essential for growth and change. Trying things and experimenting requires it. There is no other way to do it. You can sometimes choose which discomfort you want, but you cannot choose to have none.

It's ok (and totally normal) to want change and at the same time want to avoid discomfort. See if you can notice and name that and work through that conflict in yourself with curiosity and self-compassion. How might the part of you that wants change, help the part of you that is trying to avoid the discomfort? How you frame this makes a difference in how you experience it. If you can drop into curiosity – great! Practice doing more of that. Next, see if you can find the thrill of figuring things out. The road won't be smooth, and you are going to have to get uncomfortable over and over and over if growth is where you want to go. To get yourself familiar with this kind of discomfort, try making a deal with yourself to sit with the discomfort. PN calls this The Ten-Minute Discomfort Deal and it goes like this:

The 10-Minute Discomfort Deal

Today, we'd like you to make a "discomfort deal" with yourself.

1. When I feel discomfort, I promise to sit with that discomfort – in whatever form it takes – for ten minutes.
2. During that time, I will notice and name the discomfort as best I can.

3. After that, I will make the choice I feel is appropriate.

Sounds doable, right? If ten minutes feels like too much, try five, or two. Start where you are and build up your tolerance for discomfort in the name of future you. As Ray Dalio says, "It's up to you to connect what you want with what you need to do to get it and then find the courage to carry it through."

Be Honest With What You Are Willing To Do

You are in charge. This is your life and your journey. You get to decide if there are things you are willing to do and not willing to do. Things you *will* give up and *won't* give up. Trade-offs you want to make and ones you won't. Going through the exercise of identifying these on paper can free you from spinning your wheels trying to change in places you just don't want to right now. It asks you to get real with what expectations are yours and what expectations belong to others (see chapter 4). All of this is about doing what matters most to you, right now. Give yourself permission to get real with that and then you can focus your energy on making changes in the places you are *actually* willing to make them. Of course, this can change over time and it's a good thing to check back in. Remind yourself as many times as you need that you are creating an Owner's Manual for *you*, in your life and your body right now. Answer these questions for yourself (remember there are no wrong answers, nothing bad is going to happen to you if you take a guess and get it wrong, I promise.):

1. What do I want?
2. What am I willing to do to get that right now?
3. What won't I do to get that right now?

You get to set the rules and choose. Always. The best way to take the struggle out of it is to step into your power here and be honest with yourself and what you really want. Consider this as you decide what you will try and experiment with. There's no point in trying something you *know* you aren't willing to do for even a little while. If it isn't clear, then try it and see. Based on what you experience, it will become clear if it is a fit for you or not.

Dip Your Toe In

A dip-a-toe-in experiment is one that allows you to sneak up on a change more cautiously and get a taste of it. This is a great approach to try in a place you are feeling a large amount of resistance (fear) that may be getting in the way of you getting started. You can also think of this as testing the edges of your comfort zone. Pros of this approach are that you are shrinking the change to a small approachable one that will allow you to feel safe enough to take it on. Consider where you might use a *dip your toe in* experiment.

Rip Off The Band-Aid

The *rip-off-the-band-aid* approach is just like it sounds; you go all in and see what comes. This is a bolder approach that is better in some circumstances for some people but not necessarily for everything and everyone. You may subconsciously feel there is a sense of bragging rights in doing things this way (the old "I did it cold turkey" kind of thing). Check your expectations and remember you are looking to play the long game. You may find this is a great approach when dropping an old story or identity you have about yourself and it is time to move on from old you. See if you can rip-off-the-Band-Aid and let it go (without leaving claw marks all over it). As you consider your next experiment, where might a *rip off the band-aid* approach work for you?

Cycle In And Out Of Difficult Changes

Some things you experiment with or specific types of changes you focus on will be more or less difficult for you than others. Some are less difficult in terms of time pressures (like time to add a glass of water versus adding another workout); some are less difficult in terms of emotional work (like adding a vegetable instead of chips at lunch versus adding a vegetable instead of chips in your night time snack). It can be a good idea to cycle in and out of easier and more difficult types of change versus staying in the difficult change place for a long time. What is *less* difficult to you is unique to you, and it is worth considering as you decide what to try next. Have you just come off an experiment that required some heavy emotional lifting? Does it make sense to try something a little lighter next? Or has the thrill of figuring that tough one out got you inspired to tackle another biggie? This is about being kind to yourself (remember you just learned about that) and setting yourself up for the best chance of success. As you move through experiments to build your Owner's Manual, consider this as you decide your next move.

Choose The Low Hanging Fruit

What change feels clear and easy to execute for you? One that you could say, "Yeah, I totally can do that and don't mind changing it." This is your *low hanging fruit* kind of change. The advantage of these types of experiments is that they have a high likelihood of being successful, allow you to practice the process of being a *changer,* and the good feelings you get from them can inspire more action. For many, drinking more water is a great "low hanging fruit" place to start. It's easy to execute, you can prime your changing muscle, figure out the pace of change that works for you, and experience the thrill of solving a problem.

Find The Log Jam To Unlock More Change

A practice or change you make that has a positive domino effect on a bunch of other things is a *log jam* type of change. If you clear this one blockage out, other things will run more smoothly. Experimenting with more or better quality sleep is a change that fits in here. When sleep improves, cravings for sugary foods settle down, you are clearer and better able to regulate your emotions, which helps you to eat the way you intend to. *Phew!* That's a lot of positives that flow out of one specific change. Where might you have a log jam going on? What is one change you could try that might create a flood of positive changes as a result?

Do The Thing Before The Thing

To make your change strategic, pick what seems like the logical next step in the progression. An easy example to prime your progression thinking is to consider the steps in learning to run. To learn to run, you must first learn to walk. To learn to walk you must first be able to stand. To learn to stand, you must first have the strength to sit. You get the idea. It's not uncommon for us as adults to skip steps and try to go right to the running. The sequence of steps in a nutrition change progression is not always as clear as the running example, but often it is less complicated than you lead yourself to believe it is. You help your clients through small steps. See if you can put your coaching hat on for yourself. Ask yourself this: Suppose you did know what the next step was, what might it be? If you are still unclear, someone with experience in what you are working on, "outside eyes" like a coach, can save you trial and error time by helping you see the next step faster. Ask yourself, "Is it possible that I am missing a step here? Is there something that might come before this that would smooth this out or make it less difficult?" Krista Scott-Dixon calls it, "The thing before the thing." If the leaps are too big or you skip a step, you may find it doesn't work, and it's not because you're heading in the wrong direction, it's simply because there was a step that was missed. Think about the thing before the thing. Ask yourself, "Is there a step in this process that makes sense to do before I do this?"

Evaluate

You've decided what to try and you're willing to try it, now it's time to decide how to evaluate it. At the end of the day, what you want to know is, "How's this working for me?" Think about evaluating not just the impact on your body but the impact on your life. All things that work to move you towards your health, performance, and/or body composition goals, may not work for your life (and vice versa). Prepping and cooking meals from scratch each day and eating each one of them sitting at the table may work for fat loss but it may not work for your job, your kid's evening soccer practice, and when you travel each week for work. There are endless numbers of things you could measure but to make your evaluation is meaningful; connect what you measure to what matters to you.

You will likely feel a pull to make this complicated. Shoot to simplify it instead. Reflecting and journaling on the basic but powerful question, "How's this working for me?" may be all you need. In some cases, gathering data from your experiments will be necessary for you to answer this question. Sorting and gathering data in a meaningful way will allow patterns and other useful information to emerge. I will give you some tools for that here and you can pick and choose which ones are a fit for how *you* work.

A note about choice before we move forward. You are not obligated to take action on anything you learn in this process. Read that again. The truth is, as you collect information and learn about yourself, what you do with the information you collect and the things you learn about yourself is 100 percent up to you. You can change something, you can change nothing. Release judgment from this. These are both actual and valid choices that are yours to make. Not your partners or your parents or your friends. Yours. Just because you've discovered something does not mean you *have to* change it right now, or ever. You are an adult and it is still your life (just like it was when you first started reading this book). Align your actions with what matters most to you – whatever that looks like - that's what this is all about. *Your* Owner's Manual.

You want to put your awareness curiosity and compassion to work in evaluation. Here are some other principles to consider:

Put Your Scientist's Hat On

If it helps to actually put a hat on … or a lab coat … or pull out a microscope, go for it! Do what you need to get in the mood. In the right frame of mind. The more you can look at this information like data with a non-judgmental, inquisitive process, the more accurate of an assessment you will have of what you see (it can even get a little fun)! Get your curiosity going. When you find the thrill in discovering and finding solutions to problems, you can move from saving joy for the outcome to enjoying the ride.

Capture *Meaningful* Progress

So much change happens under the surface. When I did my year with a nutrition coach, I ended the year at the same weight I started. Sure, there were fluctuations but at the end of it, I didn't lose a pound. My body composition sure did change though (photos and the way my clothes fit showed me that) and I've seen this again and again with clients (you likely have too). If weight were my only metric, I could have considered the year a failure. The reality is, the massive amount of change that happened *in* me lead to my year being a huge success. It was *that* change that allowed me to get my eating (and life) back in alignment - the weight then took care of itself. So how do you measure that? Widen the scope in terms of what you measure. Think about your goal and what else matters to you, and measure that too. How will you know if the thing you're trying out is working for you? How can you measure that? Get creative starting with what *matters* and working back from there.

Tracking your progress or changes is helpful to keep you engaged with the change, too. Your human instinct will have you on to the next thing without even pausing a beat to see where you've come from, or recognizing and celebrating small changes. There is value in looking down to see how far you've climbed and having data to help you do that. Progress happens in all kinds of places that have nothing to with the relationship of your mass with gravity.

Record It

Scientists record data, and that is a good idea for you too. Write it down somewhere, use your phone, a spreadsheet, or tracking sheet. A record is valuable for a number for reasons, but two big ones, in your case, are these:

1. **You will forget (you are human)**. Grab a paper right now and write down everything you had to eat or drink in the last twenty-four hours including the times you ate and where you were and who you were with. Okay, how'd you do? Do you think you got it all? Like, *really* got it all? Imagine as a scientist you told your boss you didn't record the data because you have a great memory. Right. It's not like you're evaluating microscopic organisms in a petri dish that are going to develop a new type of plastic. You're talking about your *life* here. Let's do all we can to get this right. Lovingly

acknowledge your humanness, and *write it down*. You don't have to record everything forever in the most specific detail. Think about the data and info you need right now, and record what is *relevant* to that. For instance, if your focus is eating more veggies, does it serve you to weigh and measure every morsel of everything you eat in a day? Of course not. Track your veggie intake. You get it. Focused recording. Get the data you need to make the next decision to build out that section of your Owner's Manual. Simplify and leave the rest for another time.

2. **You are a creature of habit (you are human)**. It's all about the patterns. Recorded data can bring to light patterns in your behavior that you may not have known were there before. They are so familiar to your brain, that if you try to process these *in* your brain alone, it makes your job a lot harder. Identifying patterns for yourself works best when you can look at the data in front of you to evaluate it.

A note about recording and consistency. How many times have you had a client who recorded every detail in MyFitnessPal or an elaborate spreadsheet without ever looking back at the data? They tell you, "Recording it keeps me on track." Recording is not just about the data but about the *act* of recording. What's that really about? Pause. The power is in the pause. What does the act of recording cause you to do? Right. To record during the day, you have to *pause* to do it. If you're recording at the end of the day, you have to *pause* to reflect on it. In that pause, the magic happens. You disrupt the pattern of behavior that you've followed in a default way for a long time (maybe your whole life), you give yourself a moment to pull out of a possible emotional decision and tap into our intentions. You get to look at choosing between what you want now and what you want most. Many good reasons to record. Give it a try and see how it works for you.

Find Your Bright Spots

Bright spots are the places where things are working well. It's human nature when you're trying to solve a problem to look at where things are going wrong and try to fix that. Make sense, right? You want to fix it so you focus on where you think it's broken. There is a place for that but a far better approach to lasting change is to focus on the where things are going *right*. Your bright spots. Look at where you did do the thing you intended to do. Where you ate the veggie, you got to the gym, you paused before you ate, you slowed down. Ask yourself, "What is different here? What is unique about this that allows it to work better?" Jerry Sternin called these "bright spots" which he explained as "observable exceptions recognized as producing results above the norm with only the same kinds of resources". Part of the beauty of this focus is that it recognizes that sustainable solutions are *already* in use. You are already doing things that are working somewhere which means you already have the skill and resources you need to make those things happen and get the outcome you desire. Let's shine a light on what's already working and clone that in as many places as possible.

In your evaluation, become a miner for bright spots. Use that as a starting point for change. Look at what *is* working and ask yourself how you can do more of that.

Here are some questions to begin to tune your bright spots radar:

- What seems to help me do X?
- In an average day, let's see if I can find the places I seem to be most successful.

- During the hour before I feel motivated to eat well, what happens? What are all the steps?
- How can I do more of that (the things that are already working well for me)?

Make Use Of Believable Others

One of the inconveniences of being human is that you are not able to see all things about yourself all the time. You have blind spots about yourself (covered in Chapter 4). The sooner you accept that there are things you don't know or can't see, the better your chances to begin seeing them. In order to see these things – which is a great idea if you really want to nail this change process and claim back your life – you will at times have to listen to, and reflect on, observations from others. If you and another person have opposable views about something, chances are that one of you is wrong. As you are evaluating, it's worth finding out if the one who has it wrong is you. The trick here is it can't be just any others. In the book *Principles*, Ray Dalio talks about finding *believable others* to help you on this path. Ask yourself, "How believable is this person giving their opinion?" Dalio defines believability like this: "Believable people are those who have repeatedly and successfully accomplished the thing in question—who have a strong track record with at least three successes—and have great explanations of their approach when probed." Seek out and consider the input of believable others as you evaluate. Especially in places you feel stuck, listen openly with the desire to know the truth.

Decide Based On Data You Know

Even when you feel like you have nothing to go on, you always have some data to work with. The ideal version of *data* you may be looking for is data that shines a beacon on exactly what you need to do and where you need to go next. The reality is that life doesn't work that way. Sometimes (often), you have an endless number of next steps to consider and no clear way to know which one is right. You don't need to know which is right, you need to decide which one you want to try next. This is a place where you are at risk of getting stuck in inaction or continuing to do the thing you know isn't working. So don't do that anymore. Try something, *anything,* that is not that thing and suddenly you're on the path to figuring it out. Imagine you are living in a city that you *know* you don't want to live in. The possibilities of where you could move to are endless (anywhere else in the world), and you don't know where to go. You feel like you need more info about other possible cities to decide. So you set out to research the pros and cons of other cities but can't seem to settle on the right one. While you are thinking and trying to decide where to move, you end up living in the place you *know* you don't want to be in for another ten years. You are no further ahead than you were. You have no new experiences to help inform your decision. Use the data you have. You know you don't want to be here, so try somewhere else. It doesn't have to be the perfect somewhere else, but chances are you will learn more about where you do want to be with the experiences you gather along the way. You've given yourself an opportunity to collect more data. Experience feeds clarity more powerfully than thinking does. Experience your way to the answer.

What Data To Collect

Now you have principles to apply in how you evaluate the data you have. Let's talk about what data you may want to collect that is specific to eating and weight management. Here are some to consider:

Weight

Your relationship with the scale is a personal one that is closely tied to expectations. That relationship can often look like this: if the number is down, it's a good day, your mood picks up, and suddenly everything starts to go your way. A lower number on the scale may result in a day where you eat better, feeling motivated by your success, or it may result in a day where you *reward* yourself with a little leniency for a few more discretionary calories.

The scale going up is a field day for your inner mean girl – a free-for-all of self-berating of all kinds about how bad you are, how you're never going to be able to do this, and suddenly you are the not only terrible at weight loss, you are a terrible parent, partner, professional, and person, too. *Ouch!*

The scale is a tool of measurement. Data. Let's check in with expectations. You know the half a pound to one pound of weight loss per week metric comes from a formula. It helps to have a standard to use as a guidepost. It also hurts when that number messes with your expectations in a negative way. Your body can't read formulas. It didn't get the memo that this is what the textbook said weight loss is supposed to look like. It's going to do its own thing. And your body's thing is going to be different from anyone else's body's thing anywhere ever. Read that again – it's important.

What is true of all bodies anywhere ever? They can change. They do change in response to the actions you take consistently over time.

What is true of scales? They give data. It is not the only data or even the most important data, but it is data that gives you a clue as to where you are on the path and where something may need to be tweaked. Imagine for a moment that you could wake up tomorrow and the scale would show you the number you've always dreamed of. You would step on that scale, and it would flash that number. Now imagine nothing else had changed. Same level of energy. Same ability to move. Same size of clothing. How important is that number? Is it really the most important thing? Steve Maraboli (a speaker, author, and behavioural scientist) shares a reminder of what a scale is designed measure: "[t]he scale can only give you a numerical reflection of your relationship with gravity. That's it. It cannot measure beauty, talent, purpose, life force, possibility, strength, or love. Don't give the scale more power than it has earned. Take note of the number, then get off the scale and live your life. You are beautiful!"

Be aware, curious, and compassionate about your relationship with the scale and use this metric (or don't) in a way that works best for you.

Girth measurements

Taking girth or circumference measurements can be a pain to get efficient at doing. But, boy, can they be a powerful way to measure change in your body. I can't count the number of times these measurements showed significant change when the scale didn't. This is why I encourage you to think about taking measurements for yourself. Contact me and I'm happy to share a measurement guide with you.

Photos

Like measurements, photos can be a powerful tool to show progress. When you look in the mirror at yourself each day, gradual change is not clear. You easily feel all the effort you are making, and it feels like the same face staring back at you. You're also looking through the lens of the stories in your head (which may be due for a re-write – more on that later). Consider front, side, and back photos if body composition change is something that is important to you. No one else has to see them but you. My bets are you will be glad you took them.

Tracking (and accountability)

Tracking gives you data needed to evaluate your experiments, but it also helps to keep you accountable to yourself. Think about what you need help being accountable in, and find a way to track that even if you never refer back to it again. The key here is that this works best if you use a system that allows you to track throughout the day in the moment you are taking the action you want to track versus sitting down at the end of the day and remembering back on what you did. The reason for this is the pause. Oh that glorious pause. Like you read about in the *record it* section earlier, when you stop to track, you insert a moment of pause and awareness. You may find you make a different choice than you would have if you were not pausing to track. It's a simple yet powerful tool.

Food journal

Food journals. You've seen them. In all shapes and sizes. Elaborate spreadsheets, online tracking lists, written in a notebook or on napkins. To make your food journal most helpful get clear on what exactly you're keeping the journal for. Connect it with the one thing you're working on at the time and structure your tracking to gather useful information about that. If your focus is on how you are eating and you are tuning into *hunger and fullness* cues, track that. If you're looking at *where* you're eating and how that impacts your choices, track that. Photo food journals can be a great way to get a visual look at what you eat in a day and sometimes that's all you need to see the bright spots and the gaps. Here are some questions to ask yourself:

- What one thing am I focusing on right now? (e.g. How slowly I'm eating? Lean protein rich foods? Water? My 3:00 p.m. snacking?)

- What would be useful information for me to see/know about this?
- What patterns or default paths do I think may come into play here for me?
- How can I capture that?

Part III:
Reset

Chapter 7:

Eat Better – Five Steps to Reset Your Eating

"The most powerful tool you have to transform your health is your fork."
– Dr. Mark Hyman

"Better" is different than optimal, ideal, or best. To be successful at "better" all you need to do is be better than you are right now. You don't have to perfect or even really great, you just need to be one tiny step further along the path in order to call it a success. Seems manageable, right? Yes, manageable. Not exactly sexy or inspiring. Manageable is not something you want to text home about or post on Instagram (well, unless you're me, I guess). Yet, string a whole bunch of successful "betters" together, and suddenly you're doing a *whole* lot better and your results will speak for themselves.

With eating, *better* means *basics*. When you're the expert and know your stuff, it's easy to feel the pull towards fancy ratios, complicated meal plans, and optimizing superfoods. At the same time, you know that's not where the magic is. The magic is executing your basics like a Rockstar – consistent and persistent, day in and day out, defining your basics through the lens of building your Owner's Manual with what works for you. Complicating things just makes things… complicated. Life will do a great job of that all on its own without any help from you (thank you very much). Go ahead and mess around with the fancy stuff if that's your jam; just don't let it get in the way of executing your basics. The results you want and your way through that is in the basics.

Improve Health, Performance, And Body Composition … All At The Same Time

Let's get on the same page about the definition of *good* nutrition. When you're eating well and taking care of your body with food, these three pieces are looked after: health, body composition, and performance.

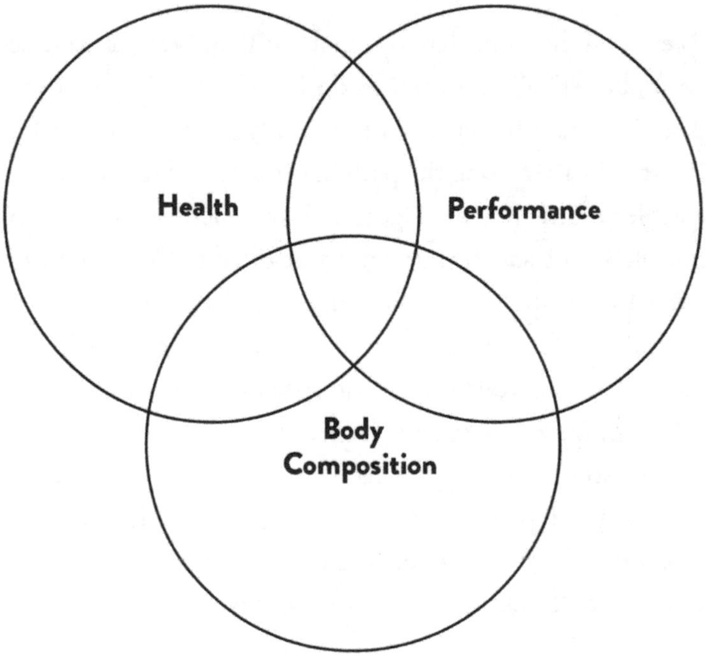

You know you've got your eating on point when it fosters improvement in *all* three areas – at the same time. Let's say you want fat loss for example (so you don't have to buy another wardrobe), that's a body composition goal. You could achieve that (in the short term) by going all-in on a restrictive crash diet, but your health (like nutrient and hormone levels) and your performance (like focus and energy at work and at home) would suffer. That's not good or sustainable nutrition in the short term or in the long run. As you build the eating section of your Owner's Manual, consider these three domains and ask yourself if you are in the happy middle place of good nutrition.

Five Steps To Reset Your Eating

If the results are in the basics, what *are* the eating basics anyhow?

ba•sics
/ˈbāsik/
noun
the essential facts or principles of a subject or skill.

What would happen if you put a bunch of health and nutrition experts who follow different eating styles and philosophies in one room together? Keto versus vegan versus Atkins versus Mediterranean. Intermittent fasters versus six-meal-a-dayers. It would make for a lively (and entertaining) debate, that's for sure. Each individual would passionately highlight the benefits of their approach and downplay the gaps or drawbacks. Human nature would drive the emphasis to what sets one way of eating *apart* from the others. But suppose you switched the lens to focus on what is the *same*. You hunted for the bright spots that unify the seemingly divergent points of view. What would emerge as key foundational practices? The basics.

There are about a million and one ways to teach the essentials of eating well. You likely have a system of your own. Here, I'm going to show you mine. Not because I'm arrogant enough to believe I have it all figured out. But because I have spent years gleaning and gathering and learning - through experience, and from other smart nutrition folks – and I've distilled that down into five steps that work for me and my clients.

Step 1: Why - Know Why You're Eating

Step 2: How - Slow Down And Leave Some Room

Step 3: Where - Eat Where You Eat Best

Step 4: What - Get Your Basic Plate In Shape

Step 5: When - Eat When You Are Hungry

As you make your way through the five steps, keep mindful of your expectations, ownership, and action:

1. Shrink the distance between where you are and where you think you should be.
2. Move from using external drivers and rules to internal values and guidelines.
3. Close the gap between knowing and doing.

Deliberately hone your focus on each of these steps, one at a time. Use them to guide what to look at in your own eating and build out that section of your Owner's Manual as you go. Experiment with the intention of finding out what pieces matter most to *you.* If you know which actions have the greatest impact on *your* goals, you will know what actions to make your foundation habits and you can choose to direct more of your energy there. Get curious. Try stuff. You want to find out what those things are.

When you go through the exercise of focusing in on each basic step, you may be surprised to find that you're a lot less consistent than you believe (oh, hello human friend). The good news in learning this is that you don't have to get fancy and complicated (phew), just get consistent and persistent in the actions that matter most *for you.* Not the ones that matter most for your friend, or colleague, or your most successful client, or the latest published researcher. You know this stuff. I know you do; I did, too. But when I really tuned in with a beginner's mindset, I was doing *some* of these steps, but I wasn't doing them in *any* kind of consistent way. Focus on building *your* Owner's Manual and follow the instructions you write - the rest will take care of itself.

Reset Step 1: Why - Know Why You're Eating

Why you eat is often overlooked. It's first because it's important. Really important. If you know why you are eating, a whole bunch of other things seem to make sense and snap into alignment. It's simple but not easy so bring your self-compassion along for the ride.

Let's start with a little exercise to focus your curiosity lens on your *whys*. Grab a piece of paper and write *Why Do I Eat?* at the top. Set a timer for three minutes and fill the paper with as many reasons you can think of to answer that question. Now, put the page aside for a minute and let's break this down.

Types Of Hunger

Hunger seems pretty simple, right? You are either hungry or you're not. Where it gets messy is the *type* of hunger. Consider three different types of hunger:

1. **Stomach hunger**. Physiological hunger. Hunger in the true sense of the word. Your body needs food for biological reasons.
2. **Head hunger**. You *think* you need to eat based on some external criteria or cue or you're hungry because you have a learned behaviour to eat in this given situation. This one can be tricky but if you pause to ask yourself, "Do I actually need food for biological reasons?" The answer is, "No." Examples include 7:00 AM is breakfast time or when I go to the movies, I eat popcorn.
3. **Heart hunger**. Emotions and feelings that are *not* stomach hunger can be experienced as hunger in the body. When something else is going on (stressed, bored, lonely, tired, irritated), you can feel the pull to eat but what you actually may need is nourishment of some other kind (a hug, a quiet moment, a chat with a friend, fresh air, journal).

Now, grab that *Why Do I Eat?* page and go through each item one by one and mark each as stomach (a plate), head (a smiley), or heart (a heart) hunger. What do you notice? Do you see a lot of hearts? Cue the curiosity and compassion.

The biggest step in getting a handle on the types of hunger is to notice and name. Use the pull to eat as a trigger to pause. Make it a practice to pause before you eat and ask yourself, "Am I hungry?

What type of hunger is this? What else might be going on for me right now?" Get curious. Based on those answers, you can choose what to do. Notice I said, "Choose." You *can* know it is not stomach hunger and choose to eat anyway. Food may solve the problem (distract or sooth you from whatever you are feeling) in the moment even though you know it is not the best solution long term. You get to decide if and when you want to try a different solution – it's your call. Start with noticing and then take it from there.

The Pull, The Pause, And The Path

Tune into this sequence. Feel the *pull* towards a behaviour or an action, insert a *pause*, and then choose your *path*. It may not feel like much, but you have taken a big first step in changing a pattern for yourself just by noticing it and calling it out (your *notice and name* superpower in action). With awareness, you bring *choice* into the equation.

You can feel the pull towards a behaviour, but you don't *have* to go there. I imagine this type of change as standing at the head of a worn path in a field of tall grass. The well-worn path is the *easy* choice. It's right there – clear as day. You know it well. For so long you have likely followed that path without even thinking about it.

Now that you *see* this path, when you find yourself at the head of it, or even partway down it, you may pause just long enough to notice where you are. You may say to yourself "I know where this path leads. I know how this ends."

In that moment, you allow yourself a choice. You may choose to continue on the path you know, or you may choose to step into the long grass and trek out a *new* path. It is unfamiliar and unclear right now and you don't know where it leads, but you *do* know where the other path leads, and you know you don't want to go there. It's an unknown and you feel fear, but you may do it, anyway. Each time you get to choose. Just because you choose the new path this time, doesn't mean you have to choose it forever. *Each* time you get to choose.

With enough passes along a new path, the old one will begin to grow over and fade and the new one will become clearer. It takes time and consistency and the first many passes require you to deliberately take the harder road. You have taken the first essential step toward a new path - *see* the path. Suppose you wanted to take a different path one of these times, what might that look like?

The Wave

Emotions are felt in the body like a wave. If you feel the rise of hunger come on suddenly that is a good clue that the "hunger" you are feeling is likely not stomach hunger. Stomach hunger tends to come on more gradually.

Emotions are felt like wave. They rise. They peak. And then they come down. When you eat in response to a wave of emotion, you're usually eating on the upside of the wave as the feeling is intensifying - before it has had a chance to peak. By doing this you don't have the experience of the full cycle of the wave to know that it will peak and then subside. This whole process can happen in as little as ninety seconds. When you feel the pull, try setting a timer to see if you can wait the wave out progressively longer each time. Practice tolerance to that wave of emotion and learn through experience that it is totally survivable.

Reset Step 2: How - Slow Down and Leave Some Room

Your speed of eating impacts your digestive health, how satisfied you feel, and how much you eat. When you eat quickly, it's easy to overshoot your needs. It takes time for your body to sense your level of fullness and give you signals to stop. While eating quickly, you can easily eat past the "we're good now" signal and land yourself at the "unbutton your pants now" or "go crash on the sofa now" signal. Slowing down gives you time to tune into your hunger and fullness levels (which you may need to relearn if eating quickly has been your M.O. for a while), feel more satisfied with your meal, and allow your digestive process the time it needs to do its job fully.

Your speed of eating also impacts your enjoyment of meal time. Is eating a chore and a stressful frenzied mess? Or is it a calm ritual of nurturing yourself – a quiet moment alone or social time shared with the people you care about? Shifting *how* you eat is a powerful way to make a difference in more than just your weight.

Slow Down

The next time you sit down to eat (or are standing at the counter to eat, or sitting at your desk to eat), set a stopwatch and see how long it takes you to finish your meal. The first time I did this, it was five minutes. *Five minutes* to eat an entire plate of food. Boy, was that a wakeup call. When I teach clients about the importance of slowing down, I see the massive difference it makes for them and yet there I was completely ignoring the speedometer for myself. I think I just assumed it wasn't an issue for me – a blind spot perhaps – until I timed myself. Then there was no unseeing that! If you suspect you are good in this department, I encourage you to confirm it for yourself by timing a few meals and getting some data.

Slowing down *sounds* like such a simple thing to do. It is simple but not easy. Why?

It's a habit

Eating quickly may be a habit you've had for a long time. Like any habit it will take some time and deliberate practice to learn to slow down. You are squeezing food into short windows between meetings at work or running kids to soccer practice or just generally fitting all the things that you have to get done in a normal day. Getting this eating thing over with, because you can, seems like a great place to gain back a few extra minutes. You adapted to what you needed and it met the need you had at one time. Or maybe it never really served you but you were able to get away with it. Your body is now telling you that can't get away with it anymore. It isn't serving you now.

It's coping

Eating is a coping and numbing strategy, so slowing down and tuning in may suddenly make other problems feel more acute. *Gulp*. That's not easy stuff. When your head and heart are full of noise and problems to solve, a quiet moment with yourself, tuning in, can be uncomfortable. *Very* uncomfortable. Eating quickly gives you a great distraction to distance yourself from that discomfort. Knowing that may not make it any easier, but it may reset your expectations and leave a little room for self-compassion. Go easy on yourself as you build this skill. This also calls you to get super deliberate about your slow down game.

Many of the strategies on awareness in Chapter 5 apply well to tuning in to your eating. Here are a few more effective ones specific to eating:

1. **Set a timer**. Ideally, twenty minutes to eat your meal is the magic number to shoot for. As always, start where you are. Add two or three minutes to your baseline eating time and go from there. Hint: It worked better for me to use a stop

watch counting *up* to twenty minutes versus a timer counting down. Somehow the countdown had me feeling like I was racing to the finish line (not helpful when you are trying to slow down!)

2. **Put your utensils down between bites**. Like, right down. Let go of those puppies and put them on the table. You can do it, I know you can.
3. **Chew and swallow the food in your mouth before you put the next bite in**. You may be surprised to find you are putting your next mouthful in before the last one is cleared.
4. **Count the number of chews**. See how many times you are currently chewing your food and increase that a few chews at a time.
5. **Single-task your eating**. How many other things do to do while you are eating? Book open, work out, computer on, phone scrolling, up and down from the table (if you are sitting at all). It is pretty tough to tune in with all those distractions. When you're eating, go all in and see what happens.
6. **Have a pleasant conversation while you eat.** When you have someone to share a meal with, breathe, chat, and enjoy the company. Give yourself a good reason to want to slow down and hang out a while.

Leave Some Room

Eating slowly allows you to fine tune when you choose to stop eating. Creeping weight gain is a sign that you've consistently been eating more than your body needs so it's time to try it a different way. It will take some time to relearn what different levels of hunger and fullness feel like for you – slowing down is key. It is really difficult to tune into these if you are racing through your meal. Without realizing it, I had spent so much time ignoring my hunger signals that I had no idea what they truly felt like when I deliberately started this practice. Then I got curious, "Well, if not using hunger and fullness, what are my clients and I using to determine when to stop eating?" Here's what I discovered:

A clean plate

Raise your hand if you are a member of the clean your plate club. Yup, me too. That was the number one thing I was using to determine when to stop eating – an empty plate meant I was done (or made room for me to go back for a second plate and then eat *that* one until I was done). If you think about a child or younger you, it likely makes sense where this comes from. You grew up in a home where "wasting" food was not tolerated and that message is ingrained in your DNA. Your parents worked hard to put food on the table and there are children in _____ (insert other part of the world) starving right now! Clean your plate. Perhaps it was something else? In your life, at some point, you learned that if there is food on your plate you are to keep eating until it's gone and you are *bad* if you don't.

A portion you *should* have

You are following recommendations from a food guide or a diet book or what someone else is doing. You portion the prescribed amount and you eat that. Sometimes it's too much, sometimes it's not enough. Either way, the data you have (your creeping weight) tells you this strategy is missing the mark.

You can't eat another bite

Your learned endpoint to a meal is a screaming sense of fullness. When you are stuffed and can't eat another bite, you stop. It's easier to *feel* hunger and fullness at the extremes – *really* hungry or *really* full. In-between is the murky middle. It's less clear and it takes tuning in (slowing down) and deliberate practice to find your way around that middle ground. Suppose your desire to feel that sense of fullness comes from somewhere, where might that be? Is there an underlying fear of going hungry that stems from a time in your life when you did not have enough food? As a child? Or as a broke student? Perhaps you made an unconscious vow to yourself that once you had the means, you would make sure to never feel hungry again? Or you would get to reward yourself with the gift of eating as much delicious food as you want.

Perhaps fullness equals security. Perhaps there is a void or *emptiness* in you that you may be trying to fill with food (*Gulp*)? Perhaps it's something else? You know from your own experience working with clients that often (most) times it's not just about the food. You are here because you want to move through this and feel back in alignment. As difficult as it may be to consider these things, it is worth reflecting on to see if there may be a blind spot you are missing or something you are pretending not to see. Something else under the surface that may be at play. If there is, awareness is the first step forward and it creates room for you to begin to sort through it, should you choose to.

As you reflect on the cues you use to signal you are done eating, consider if they are external cues or internal cues. Are you using something outside of you to guide your decision when to stop (like a clean plate or a prescribed portion)? Are you using a misaligned internal cue (like feeling *really* full)? Make note of what your default tendency is in your Owner's Manual and think about an experiment you could try to reset that cue to serve you better. The goal is to move away from external rules and *should* to drive your eating to internal cues and signals to guide your eating.

Reset Step 3: Where - Eat Where you Eat Best

I remember a time when eating in the library was a big hard *no* – the sound of a crinkling wrapper had librarians everywhere spring into full combat mode. Now we have *cafes* in the library. The food landscape has changed. Food and eating are welcome almost everywhere. You are *invited* to eat almost everywhere. I challenge you to think about a place that doesn't have food on display inviting you to grab a little snack to *solve* that hunger *problem* of yours. It's also socially acceptable for you to eat anywhere. There is a good chance the dining table in your house is primarily used for everything but dinning.

As you build out this section of your Owner's Manual, tune into *where* you eat. *Where* has a big influence on the why, how, what, and when of eating. Your *where* can support you in making the changes you want to make in your eating, or it can get in the way of those changes and make them more difficult (big time). Setting some loving guidelines for yourself about where you eat is a big vote in favour of desired future you.

Begin with awareness, curiosity, and compassion. Check in with your expectations around where you eat (hint: if you think you are immune to the impact of this on your choices, I urge you to take an honest closer look). Discover the places you eat best, record those in your Owner's Manual, and aim to have your meal *there* every chance you get. If you feel the pull to eat in places that are bad news for you – say standing in the line at Marshall's – see if you can ride out the wave. Hunger is not an emergency - even though every food marketer on the face of the earth would like you to believe it is. Instead of having to call on yourself to make a decision *each* time, create a list called "Where I Will Eat" in your Owner's Manual. Enjoy your food there and when the food calls to you in a place other than the ones in your Manual, the answer is, "This is not a place I eat." and you get to move along. Questions to reflect on:

- Where do I eat my best? Where am I most likely to eat slowly and mindfully the way I intend to eat? How can I do more of that?
- Where do I get into trouble with eating? Where do you find it most difficult to eat the way you intend to? Where are my red-light eating places?
- What loving guardrails will help me eat where I eat best?

Reset Step 4: What - Get Your Basic Plate in Shape

You may be surprised that *what* is this far down the list. What you put into your mouth is of course important, you know that. I purposely address the *why, where,* and *how* first because what you eat is heavily influenced by those other factors. By making small (or big) improvements in the first three steps, there is a really good chance you will have made improvements in *what* you are eating without any deliberate focus on doing that (bonus). Digging into the details of what you eat can bring up loads of resistance and lots of opportunity to feel stuck (especially with all the info about this swimming around in your expert brain). Your inner toddler can spring to life fighting back against the feeling that changing what you eat equals taking a bunch of stuff away. A tantrum-ing inner toddler makes consistency and long term change more difficult. So let's focus on *adding* and *shifting* and *swapping* stuff versus taking stuff away, okay?

With positive changes already under way from steps one to three, you will likely land in step four with some success under your belt you can build on. You may already have a solid foundation of high-quality foods that you consume on the regular (check). You also may not (remember that being human thing?) Either way, a solid reset starts at the basics. Even if you think you've got this one down, I encourage you to gather data to confirm that for yourself and be sure you aren't missing something key (remember blind spots?) Perhaps you aren't getting *as many* vegetables in a day as you think you are? Perhaps *more* simple carbs are creeping in? Maybe protein is missing from your plate *frequently* versus occasionally? You know the drill. Put that coaching hat on and turn the lens on yourself, or get a second set of eyes to take a look for you. These kinds of oversights are not intentional, they are an inconvenience of being human (there's that *again*). If there is something here to find that's getting the way of your progress, you want to find it, right? So let's dig in.

Use Your Hands To Build Your Plate

I've tested *a lot* of different tools and nutrition approaches over my fifteen plus years as a registered dietitian. I imagine you've tried at least a few too. A good tool is one that is clear to understand, simple to follow, and allows you to gets solid, consistent results. The best approach also plays nicely with the rest of your life. Scales and measuring cups work well for some people, some of the time. For most, the less complicated the better. There will always be some grey areas that you get to sort out for yourself – like "Do I count beans as a protein or a carbohydrate?" or "Where does a mixed casserole fit?" (you've heard these questions before). The good news is, you're writing *your* Owner's Manual, so you don't have to get stuck in the details. You get to decide about the grey areas based on what works best for you. The only "rules" that matter are the instructions you have written based on what you know works for *you* (hooray!) If you've been using the same system or approach for a long while, and you suspect it may not be working fantastic for you any longer, I encourage you to experiment with something new. The *Portion Control Guide* by *Precision Nutrition* is my go to tool and that is what I will share with you here. Here are some reason I find it so effective:

1. **Portions are "measured" using your hands**. A convenient portable tool that is proportionate to your body.
2. **Vegetables are in a group all on their own**. Fruits are counted in with the carbohydrate dense foods. If you are not deliberate about getting your vegetables, you won't get them. Period. Even if you're a nutrition coach. When fruits and vegetables are grouped together, it's easy to meet your "requirement" with mostly fruit and not consistently meet that veggie quota for great health (inconvenience of being human). It's effective to call attention to this by having the veggies in their own group.
3. **The guidelines are given per meal**. You eat one meal at a time so a tool that gives you a system to build one meal at a time, eliminates extras steps of having to work back from daily totals. It may seem simple but the fewer steps between you and your desired action, the better.
4. **It works as a guide for any type of diet or style of eating**. Vegan to meat loving and everything in between. It gives you a starting point of what makes up a well-rounded plate and you adjust from there.

Portion Control Guide

The full guide and printable infographic of it can be found here: https://www.precisionnutrition.com/calorie-control-guide-infographic

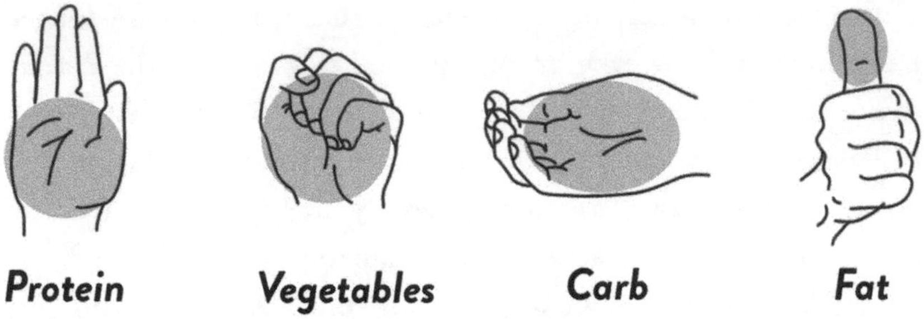

Here's how it works. Foods are grouped into the following categories: protein, vegetables, carbs, and fats.

Protein

Hand measure: Your palm (same thickness and diameter as your palm).
Foods included: Lean protein-dense foods like meat, fish, eggs, cottage cheese and Greek yogurt, beans.
How much: Men two palm-sized portions at each meal (~40-60 g protein). Women one palm-sized portion at each meal (~20-30 g protein).

Vegetables

Hand measure: Your fist (same thickness and diameter as your fist).
Foods included: Veggies like broccoli, spinach, salad, carrots.
How much: Men two fist-sized portions at each meal. Women one fist-sized portion at each meal.

Smart Carbs

Hand measure: Your cupped hand.
Foods included: Carbohydrate-dense foods like grains, starches, beans, and fruit.

How much: Men two cupped-hand sized portions (~40-60 g carbs). Women one cupped-hand sized portion (~20-30 g carbs). Note: The *smart* part is about which carbs you choose. Whole food carbohydrates are what you are going for here.

Healthy Fats

Hand measure: Your thumb.

Foods included: Oils, butters, nut butters, nuts, and seeds.

How much: Men two thumb-sized portions (~15-25 g fat). Women one thumb-sized portion (~7-12 g fat).

Note: The *healthy* fat part is about looking for less-processed and/or whole food sources of fat.

At the end of the day, men eating 3-4 meals like this would get around 2,300 to 3,000 calories each day. Women eating 3-4 meals like this would get around 1,200 to 1,500 calories each day.

If you are more active and you need more, do that. Experiment with adjusting your portions up based to get the right balance of performance and body composition goals met. Try it. Evaluate the data. Do what works for you. Record that in your Owner's Manual.

Other key elements in the "what" of eating are:

Make Water Your Beverage Of Choice

What you drink can have a sneaky but significant impact on your health and your weight. When looking at your *what*, check in with your beverages. It's not just about the soda either. Think sweetened teas and fancy coffee drinks like Frappuccinos, fruit drinks and juices, sports drinks, sweetened rice and soy and almond milks. Also think alcohol. Collect the data. How many calorie containing drinks are you actually getting each day? In a week? You may be surprised to find just how often you are getting them and just how many unwanted extra calories are sneaking into your day. It's easy to take in an extra 100 to 200 calories per day from drinks. You know the math … even if your meals are on point, these extra calories add up and voila creeping weight and pants that don't fit. Experiment with two weeks of replacing all calorie containing drinks with water or black tea and see what happens. If the thought of doing that (especially removing alcohol) throws up huge resistance in you, you may have just hit on something that is worth exploring a little further. What value are these drinks adding in your day? How are they serving you? Be aware and deliberate about the drinks you do choose to have and enjoy and aim for mostly calorie-free beverages (water, black tea, or coffee) the rest of the time. Which sugary or empty-calorie drinks could you easily switch out for water in favor of your goals?

Choose The Better Food Most Of The Time

In any given eating situation, there is a better food choice and a worse food choice. It varies widely based on what options are available to you. The *better* choice in one situation – a whole foods protein bar (better) over a highly processed chocolate bar (worse) – may be the worse choice in another situation – meal containing protein-dense lentils (better) over a whole foods protein bar (worse). It is also individual based on foods that agree with you and ones that don't. The better foods are less processed – foods closer to the way nature made them. Consider an apple for example. The whole apple would be the best choice. Moving along the continuum might be chunky apple sauce, apples sauce with sugar and cinnamon added, 100% pure apple juice, dried apple chips, apple cocktail, apple fruit roll up, apple pie, apple flavoured jelly beans (not really apple at all, right?). You get the idea. The further along the continuum you move, more nutrients are lost in the process and more things are added (salt, sugar, artificial flavours, preservatives etc). An easy question to ask yourself is, "Which option is closer to the way nature made it?"

Here are some additional criteria to consider:

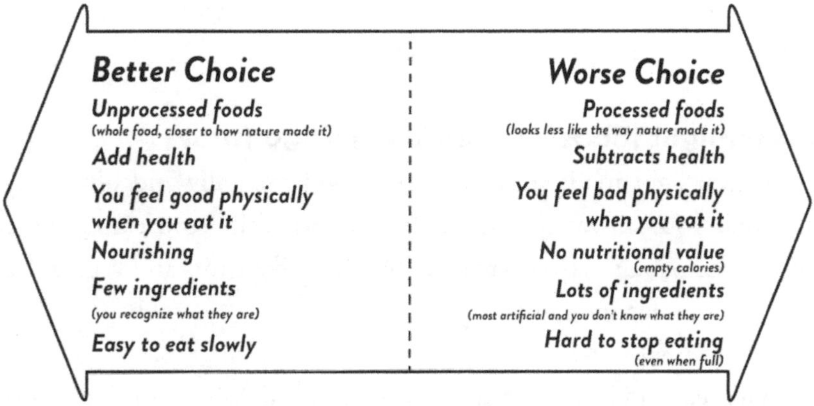
Better Choice
Unprocessed foods
(whole food, closer to how nature made it)
Add health
You feel good physically when you eat it
Nourishing
Few ingredients
(you recognize what they are)
Easy to eat slowly
Worse Choice
Processed foods
(looks less like the way nature made it)
Subtracts health
You feel bad physically when you eat it
No nutritional value
(empty calories)
Lots of ingredients
(most artificial and you don't know what they are)
Hard to stop eating
(even when full)

Make it a practice is to choose the "better food" most of the time. What most of the time is depends on the trade-offs you want to make and the body composition change you're aiming for. When you choose the occasional *worse* food, be deliberate about choosing it - pick food that you will truly enjoy (like birthday cake) and then be deliberate about slowing down and enjoying it.

Eat Your Green-Light Foods Most Of The Time

Using the better-worse continuum as a guide, create a list in your Owner's Manual of foods that work well for you and foods that don't. A stop light system works well and it looks like this:

Red-light foods – Red means "no go"

Red-light foods are just bad news for you. Maybe they make you feel sick, or they trigger you to eat too much, or you know they're an unhealthy choice for you, etc.

Yellow-light foods – Yellow means "approach with caution"

Yellow-light foods are sometimes ok, sometimes not. Maybe you can eat a little bit without feeling ill, or you can eat them sanely at a restaurant with others but not at home alone, or you can have them as an occasional treat without much trouble.

Green-light foods – Green means "go for it"

Green-light foods make you feel good mentally and physically, and that you can eat normally, slowly, and easily stop eating when you've had enough. These are usually things like fruits and vegetables, lean protein, legumes, etc.

Get real and be honest about what foods fit where for you. I love vanilla ice cream (I know, not the most exciting flavor but I'm an ice cream purist – ask me about it sometime). Vanilla ice cream is a yellow-light food for me. More than a kid-sized serving and my gut is not happy, I have a hard time eating it sanely, and crushing ice cream by the tub is not really a vote in favor of desired future me, ya know? So, instead of pretending not to know this, I step into the reality of it and love myself by not having tubs of it around. If I want some, I have to go out and get it – which makes it a deliberate choice. If I want ice cream in the house for something else, say a kid's birthday party, I will get a flavor that I'm not a fan of (like mint chocolate chip).

This list can be incredibly freeing. It can help you more easily decide what you bring home and help you navigate what foods you eat each day without having to think hard and decide about each one (more about that in the section on food environment). If it's a red-light food, it's a no. Get deliberate about when and how often you choose the yellow-light foods. When you are grabbing for something to eat, your green-light list is your go-to.

Reset Step 5: When - Eat When You are Hungry

When your goal is general health and some weight loss (you are not doing extreme exercise or looking for extreme body composition changes), specific nutrient timing is not a main priority (which is why it is Step 5). Chances are, unless your diet is god-like, any small physiological advantages there may be of eating at very specific times, will not outweigh the advantage of you eating at the times that allow you to make the best food choices for you. Use that along with what you discover works best for your body and life as your primary guiding factors. Move towards using internal cues to guide your *when* versus external ones. Eat when you're hungry, and don't eat when you're not. Positive things happen if you eat at times that you are most likely to eat the way that you intend to - a way that serves you and your goals (typically not at 10 pm while binge watching Netflix). A number of external factors influence when you eat including:

- **Your schedule.** Set break and lunch times at work, events and activities, workout or exercise times, travel, appointments etc.
- **Other people's schedules.** When you get to share your meals with family, timing is not only based on your schedule but theirs as well (a good problem to have). You may feed your kids at times you are not hungry but want to share the meal with them or perhaps you hold off on a meal until a partner comes home from work.
- **Time on the clock.** Did you grow up in a house where 7:00 am was breakfast, 12:00 pm was lunch and 6:00 pm was supper? In this case, the clock cues you when to eat, whether you are hungry or not. Or maybe you're following an eating protocol or diet that prescribes set eating times or windows (like intermittent fasting).

- **Heart and head hunger**. Refer back to the list you generated earlier and look at all the reasons you eat that have nothing to do with your biological need for food. You eat when you go to the movies or your aunt's house or because you are out with friends. In this case, emotions or learned behavior drive your when.

Get curious about when you eat. What guides you? How do you feel when you eat at different times of the day? When in the day are you most likely to eat in a way that moves you in the direction of desired future you? Moving from external cues to use internal ones takes patience and practice. Figure out what works best for your body and your life by trying stuff (surprise surprise). Place deliberate focus on *when* you eat and practice doing what works for you. Here are some tools and tips to help you along:

Use Fasting Windows To Help You

Fasting is a period of time where you abstain from all or some kinds of food or drink. You already have periods of fasting in your day now, like when you are sleeping or between your meals. *Intermittent fasting (IF)* as an eating strategy is a popular topic in the health, wellness, and fitness spaces (chance are a client of yours has asked you about it or you've looked into it yourself). There are bunch of different protocols for cycling between periods of eating and fasting (some ranging from 16 to 24 hours) but the reality is you can choose to use fasting in any way that works for you, you don't have to follow a specific protocol. Why would you want to do IF at all? Good question. *Experiments with Intermittent Fasting* is a free e-book written by John Berardi, Krista Scott-Dixon, and Nate Green that gives a solid overview of the current landscape when it comes to IF - if you would like to geek out on this stuff (https://www.

precisionnutrition.com/intermittent-fasting/benefits-of-fasting). For our purposes, I encourage you to play around with your fasting windows if:

- **Your night time fasting window is less than ten hours**. When I see a window less than ten hours in my clients, there is usually evening or night time munching going on (and you *ain't* snacking on broccoli). Setting a specific fasting window overnight as routine can help take away the need to make decision about eating at a time you are tired and highly desirable food is at your fingertips. I like to think of this as loving yourself with a fast after ____ pm.
- **The idea of having a period in your day where you don't have to make food decisions is attractive to you**. When I was feeling stressed about my creeping weight and what was going on with my eating, I felt like I was thinking about and making decision about food *all* the time. Having spaces in my day where I was *fasting* provided some relief and was a great way to reset. Experiment with times that you run into trouble with snacking and see how it feels to add a loving fast there for yourself. Perhaps you *fast* for three or four hours between your meals and the pull for mindless munching disappears. Or maybe you *fast* at 10:00 am on Wednesdays when you have that board meeting that includes donuts and fancy coffee drinks that you have a hard time saying no to.
- **You could use some practice getting comfortable with hunger**. There is no better way to increase your tolerance to feeling hunger than to feel it on a regular basis, and know you will survive. If you're used to eating at the first sign of hunger and grazing your way through the day is not serving you, deliberate fasting is worth a try. Start where you are and gradually increase the time. If you're normally grabbing for

something else to eat an hour after your meal, try extending that to one and a half or two hours and see what happens.

The Best Number Of Meals Is The Number That Works For *You*

Eating three to four times per day tends to work best for most people but it is worth getting curious about. Drop all the *shoulds* you have around *when* to eat and allow what works for you to be your guide. Breakfast is a meal you may have a lot of *shoulds* around. I remember early in my career, the recommendation was to have something to eat within an hour of waking up. That myth that your metabolism slows if you don't or you can *boost* your metabolism if you do, is still hanging on strong. Should you have breakfast even though you don't feel like it? Try it and see. How do you feel when you have breakfast versus when you don't? Is there any change in meals in the rest of your day based on what you do? What happens to the measures that matter most to you?

Take a close look at snacks *between* meals and see if they really serve you. You may eat three to four *meals* per day but you are *actually* eating more times than that in your day. Be honest with yourself. If what you have in between meals is getting you into trouble, you want to know and find a different strategy. The types of foods you tend to grab as snacks are often not the most nutritious. Is telling yourself you "should' have snacks a loophole to give yourself permission to eat a less nutritious food? Step into the reality that you are a grown up and you can choose to eat less nutritious food any time you want, you don't need a loophole to do it.

Hunger Is Not An Emergency

Don't fall victim to the idea society has created that you have to get food *now!* You know the science. Play around with your hunger threshold. Reset your expectations around hunger so they serve you.

Questions for Reflection - Eating

Start Here

Where am I starting from? How does my eating impact my performance, health, and body composition? How are my basics right now (why, how, where, what, when)? How is my consistency with them? Where am I most consistent? Least consistent? What are my expectations about my eating? What am I doing now? What do I believe about what I "should" be doing? How can I make my expectations work for me? What stories do I tell myself about eating? What ideas do I carry with me from childhood about food and eating? Are they actually true? How do they serve me? How can I rewrite this story?

Get Curious

When do I seem to be most successful with my eating? What helps me to eat the way I intend to? How can I do more of that? What gets in the way of me eating the way I intend to? How can I clear away some obstacles? What patterns do I see in my day, week, month, year? Which patterns still serve me? Which patterns no longer serve me?

Try Stuff

What kind of experiment do I want to do right now (e.g. dip a toe in or rip off the band aide)? How will I lean into the discomfort of this? How will this make a difference? Instead of feeling __ way about __, I would like to feel __. How will this be meaningful? How will I know if it is "working" for me?

Chapter 8:

Boost Energy - Move and Sleep like Your Life Depends on It

"A good laugh and a long sleep are the two best cures for anything."
- Irish Proverb

You already know movement and sleep are important. Eating better will have the biggest impact on your weight reset but sleep and movement are key when it comes to vitality and living in alignment with what you teach. This chapter is less about the details of quality movement and sleep and more about reminding you of their importance and guiding you to experiment to make sure they have a place in your Owner's Manual.

Movement

I use the word "movement" here instead of "exercise" on purpose. What it's really about is movement. All kinds of movement. It's about being a person who values and loves themselves with movement. You don't need to have "workouts" or "programs" to move. The consistency and variety of movement throughout your day is what matters most. A detailed program can be the path to specific body composition goals or to correct dysfunctional movement patterns. But finding movement that you love and will *do* consistently is what will make the biggest difference in your long-term weight and health.

As you get curious about your movement, consider the different types of physical activity you have in your day:

Activities of daily living and fun stuff

Pause to remind yourself of the number of changes that have happened in your environment since your grandparents were young, or even since you were a child, that have taken away unplanned chances to move. Elevators, escalators, movators, dishwashers, electric garage door openers, push button or automatic openers on almost every door. Think about drive-thru's and what distance is now considered walkable.

Get curious about where you make use of "conveniences" in your day and consider how "convenient" it really is to have opportunities to move *removed*. Where can you love yourself buy adding movement back into your day - every chance you get. Be the person who pulls open doors instead of pushes buttons (go ahead and open them for someone else while you're at it), who takes the stairs, who parks at the back of the parking lot. Carry your groceries to the car if you can do it without the cart. Wash dishes by hand sometimes. Use the shovel instead of the snow thrower. Walk to your mailbox instead of stopping in your car on the way by. How many times in your day can you find reasons to go up and down the stairs at home?

Get aware of opportunities for fun types of movement. The stuff you used to do when you were a kid or that you see your own kids do. Balance on the curbs for a while when you're out for a walk or skip over the sidewalk cracks. Garden or fly a kite or climb at the park instead of sitting on the bench. Play Twister. You get the idea. As you build your Owner's Manual, get curious about these things and build that love of movement back into your life.

Strength or resistance training

Your muscle mass is important for your quality-of-life, longevity, independence, and maintenance of a healthy weight. You know this. If you don't use your muscles, you'll lose them. Especially given what we just covered in point number one there's a lot less using going on. Unless you're *deliberate* about giving your muscles the love they need to stay strong or even grow, there's a pretty good chance they're being *neglected.* It wasn't too long ago that the gym was only for bodybuilders. No one would have imagined a day where the average Jo would pay to go into a big room to pick up a variety of heavy things and put them back down. Going to the gym is just *one* way to strength train. If you don't enjoy that way, explore other ways and find one you do. There are an endless number of free plans and programs and ideas online. An endless number of opportunities to get creative in your own home picking up and putting down heavy stuff. Pick one that seems remotely appealing to you (or even marginally tolerable) and try it. Do that again and again until you find one (or many) ways to love your muscles that brings you enough joy that you want to keep doing it. If being social about it is a draw for you, then do that. Find a group or a class to join with a friend or call on your bravery and go solo (perhaps you'll bring new active friends into your life). It's worth the effort.

Cardiovascular

Training your heart and getting a sweat on is worth doing to. It does help burn calories but despite what the messaging would like you to believe, you can't out run a poor diet. So, don't make your cardio about weight loss alone (or at all about punishing yourself for the cheesecake you ate yesterday). That just doesn't serve you and you deserve better. Run, ride a bike, skip, skate, swim, ski, or something else. Find the things you enjoy because long term consistency is key.

Active recovery

Our bodies thrive on gentle types of movement for recovery sometimes versus flopping on the couch for the evening all the time. Walking is probably one of the simplest ones to do because you can do it just about anywhere most of the time. Every bit counts; five minutes, ten minutes, small chunks throughout the day. Do it alone and breathe for a quite few minutes or grab a friend or a colleague and share the benefit of deliberate activity with them. A Fitbit or a pedometer can be a great motivator for this kind of thing if that's your jam. Other active recovery movement could include gentle yoga or any number of the activities mentioned in number one.

Here are some simple guidelines to give you an idea of what this might look like based on the total number of hours you spent being active each week. Aim to have some deliberate movement each day (thirty minutes or more). Start with where you are and add from there.

- 0 to 5 hours per week - 3 hours resistance, 30 minutes cardio, 1 hour active recovery, fun stuff the rest of the time.
- 5 to 10 hours per week - 3 hours resistance, 30 to 45 minutes cardio, 2 to 3 hour active recovery, fun stuff the rest of the time.
- 10 to 15 hours per week - 3 hours resistance, 45 minutes cardio, 3 to 4 hour active recovery, fun stuff the rest of the time.

Once you've found movements that you like, see if you can build a system around it to make sure it happens on a regular basis. Predict and problem solve around obstacles and crush as many as you can.

Questions for Reflection - Movement

Start Here

Where am I starting from? How much activity do I get in my day right now? What are my expectations around type, frequency, duration, intensity of movement and exercise? What am I doing now? What do I believe about what I "should" be doing?

What do I believe about myself and exercise and movement in general? Is that actually true? How can I make my expectations work for me? When is the last time I was able to consistently do that?

Get Curious

What helps me to move? How can I do more of that? What gets in the way of me moving? How can I clear away some obstacles?

Try Stuff

Experiment with type of exercise, time of day, duration, intensity. Do I like exercise alone or with others? What do I think and how do I feel *before* exercise? What do I think and how do I feel *after* exercise?

Sleep

Getting enough sleep is often overlooked in favor of busyness and driving and striving. I can't count the number times I've had a client lose weight by making changes in sleep first. You know this to. When you get enough quality sleep you generally crave less sweets, make better food choices, and move and exercise more. All good things when you're looking to reset. Getting the sleep your body craves also lifts your mood. You are less likely to be depressed, grumpy, or moody and you are more likely to be clear and focused, make better decisions, and just be a better human overall.

The more you ask of your body in terms of health, performance, and body composition, the more you want to pay attention to sleep (take a peek back at the Cost of Getting Lean Article). Generally, eight hours of sleep each night is the magic number and at least seven is the minimum to shoot for. Get curious about your sleep. Try a sleep tracker or even just recording the time you went to bed and the time you woke up. When you're having a day that feels especially *difficult* somehow, pause and ask yourself how your sleep was the night before. When you're having an especially *productive* and *focused* day pause and ask yourself how your sleep was the night before (bright spots). You may already know the answers to these questions but recording the data and having it in front of you might be just the nudge you need to take action on it. Look for patterns in your day that seem to appear based on the number of hours of sleep you had.

There's no question one of the keys to consistent high-quality sleep is a consistent transition-to-sleep or *bedtime* routine. Which makes sense right? It's pretty unrealistic to immediately go from the busyness of a full day to a sound restful slumber. Yet you ask and expect yourself to do this all the time. Work until ten minutes before bedtime, flop into bed, and wonder why you're lying in there still thinking about the book you are writing (speaking for a friend). You spend the final minutes of your day scurrying around the house tidying up, cleaning the kitchen, or planning for the next day and then just hope your brain will shut off the moment your head hits the pillow. Perhaps it is that quiet of the night that you just don't want to let go – this one used to keep me up when I know the best way to love myself would have been to just go to bed. Especially when you have young kids in the house, it can be the only time in the day you have to yourself – to not be *on*. You just want to do something you want to do and this feels like your only chance to do it (even though you can barely keep your eyes open). I get it. There is a conflict here for sure. Something to dig into and get curious about. How can the part of you that knows that sleep is what you need in the moment, help the part of you that wants to fight to stay up? How can you balance what you want *now* with what you want *more*?

The bedtime routine that works for you does not have to be complicated and overly ritualistic. It can be. But it doesn't have to be. Experiment and see what works for you. There are many variables outside of yourself that impact your sleep especially if you have young kids in your house. Be as consistent as you can as you figure this out. Be kind and patient with yourself as you go, feeling stressed about figuring out a bedtime routine is *not* going to help anything, right? Here are some strategies to try to ease your transition to bed and improve your sleep:

- **Go to bed and wake up at about the same time each day**. An inconsistent sleep schedule makes it harder on your body to get into routine. If you can get consistent about your sleep and wake up time you will likely find it easier to fall asleep and wake up when you intend to.
- **Power down the screens at least an hour before bed (computer, TV and phones)**. This one can be tough but give

it a try for one week and see what happens. You may also try some of the settings on phones and computers now that can change and darken the light at the end of the day.

- **Get your room as dark and quiet as possible.** Light tells your body it's time to wake up. Survey your room and see if you can eliminate as many sources of light as possible. Cover light from alarm clocks or other electronics in the room. Try blackout curtains.
- **Have any caffeine in your day before noon**. Caffeine can stay in your system for quite a long time and disrupted your sleep without you even realizing it. Experiment for a week with coffee in the morning and uncaffeinated drinks the rest of the day and see what happens.
- **Do a brain dump at bedtime**. Grab a paper or notebook and write anything that's in your head to clear your mind before sleep. Get it out. You can look at it in the morning (or not). Let the page hold it for you so your mind doesn't have to.

Questions for Reflection - Sleep

Start Here

Where am I starting from? How much sleep do I get on average right now? What is my range of hours of sleep? What are my expectations about quality sleep and transitioning to sleep? What am I doing now? What do I believe about what I "should" be doing? How can I make my expectations work for me?

What do I believe about myself and sleep in general? What stories do I tell myself? Is that actually true? How could I rewrite this story?

Get Curious

What helps me to go to bed and sleep well? How can I do more of that? What gets in the way of me going to bed and sleeping well? What wakes me up at night? How can I clear away some obstacles?

Try Stuff

What do I think I might like as part of a sleep routine? How can I get my environment to support better sleep?

Chapter 9:

Cultivate Environment – Create an Operating Space that Supports You

"Every cell in your body is listening to your thoughts."
- Dr. Mark Hyman

Your environment matters. A lot. Both the environment around you and the one inside you have a big impact on your ability to be consistent and persistent with your actions. The right environment can give you a boost in the direction of desired future you and the wrong one can put extra obstacles in your path. Get curious about your environment. Identify habits and patterns and look for ways to shape the path. Add instructions to shape your environment, in your favor, to your Owner's Manual.

en•vi•ron•ment
/inˈvīrənmənt/
noun
the surroundings or conditions in which a person, animal, or plant lives or operates.

External Environment

While writing this book, I worked mostly from a desk on the main floor of my home. There is a bathroom about five steps from my desk, which is convenient because I like to drink tea while I work and write, and you can guess what that means in terms of trips to the bathroom. As I dug into my writing work, I realized that I was going pretty long stretches of sitting without much movement other than the five steps to the bathroom and back. I was starting to feel it in my neck and shoulders, and I thought to myself, "Okay, time to make a plan for moving a little more." I did get up a little more the following days, but it was inconsistent at best. One day I hopped up from my desk and into the bathroom and saw that the toilet paper roll was empty. So, I ran upstairs to use the bathroom there.

The next day, I had not changed the roll and dashed in a couple more times to see it empty before I ran up the stairs. On about the fifth trip since the empty roll, I didn't even go into the downstairs bathroom at all, I went directly upstairs. When I realized what had just happened, I couldn't help but smile. Inconvenience had given me exactly what I needed to take the action I wanted to take. It was that simple but super powerful - my environment was set up to help me do what I intended to do. I did (eventually) replace the toilet paper roll but now when I'm doing a long stretch of work at my desk, I love myself with the routine of using the upstairs bathroom. It's a habit now.

The first step is to take stock. Look around. Get aware and curious. See where your environment is helping you (do more of that) and see where is making your job more difficult (get ruthless about eliminating any obstacles you can). When it comes to food, you may believe you are in solid control of all your food decisions, but your environment is a bigger influence that you realize (surprise!).

You make over 200 decisions about food each day and most of these decisions are subconscious.

You *know* you're eating environment impacts how much you eat but as a nutrition expert that is aware of this, you may trick yourself into believing that you are somehow immune *because* you know. This is so important that it is worth revisiting. You may know the work of Brian Wansink from Cornell University. He has spent years researching the impact environment has on food choices. The message that comes out time and time again in his studies is that when the environment sets you up to eat more, you eat more. Even if you know this and you try not to, you eat more. This is a good place to remind your nutrition expert self that you are human first.

Here are some key external environment changes to take a look at that can make a big difference:

Keep The Foods You Want To Eat Around And The Ones You Don't Out

Berardi's Law, from John Berardi, goes like this, "If a food is in your house, you, someone you love, or someone you marginally tolerate will eventually eat it." It's a little cheeky but oh so true. If food is in your house, it will get eaten. Think carefully about what you bring into the house and keep around you.

Set your environment up for success by keeping the foods you *want* to have *handy* and the foods you *don't want* to have *away*. Look at convenience. There are places that convenience is your foe (how close the cookie jar is or having your phone at your fingertips while working) and sometimes convenience is your friend (washed and cut veggies waiting for you in the fridge). Inconvenience can also be friend (like my toilet paper run) or foe (having to dig through a muddled pile of lids for your food storage containers when doing food prep). Visible open candy dishes or cookie jars on the counter or table or the desk at work will make you eat more without realizing it. If there are more steps between you and the chip bag, you create an extra barrier that gives you a moment to pause and think about the choice you're making. So, store them up in that high cupboard that requires you to get a chair or in the basement pantry - you get the idea. Refer to your red-yellow-green light food list and see if there are any red-light foods in your space. Decide what you want to do about that. This requires maintenance. Check in on the foods you keep around your house (and where are you keeping them) on a regular basis.

Use Smaller Plates For Smaller Portions

The size of the dishes you use matter. Here is a great video from PBS's in defence of food series that demonstrates this: www.pbs.org/video/in-defense-food-size-plate. I've become deliberate about the plate sizes in my home about over the last few years. I spent time finding the right size of dish to hold just the right portion for me of the foods I eat most often. It has been worth every bit of effort. Yes, I practice eating slowly, being all in on eating while I'm doing it, and leaving a little room, but having just that right portion amount in front of me is like a little safety net. If my old-clean-your-plate ways rear their ugly heads that day, or I'm eating distracted for one reason or another, minimal damage is done. I can't count the number of times a client of mine lost weight simply by switching to smaller plates or bowls with making little to no changes in *what* they ate.

Skip The Supersized Packages

Portion sizes create our consumption norms. When you eat from bigger packages you eat more. Period. Even *you* can't get around this one. Marketers do a fabulous job of making it feel like buying the jumbo size is great value (can you say, 'Costco'). I encourage you to get curious about this and see how much you eat when you have a big package versus when you have a small one. If you want to skip the experiment in this case and just trust the fact that the data for you is likely to show you the same thing it shows for every other human, you can save yourself a little trouble. Does upsizing meals when out, or popcorn at the movies, or all you can eat bread at dinner *really* adding value to your life? Get aware and give yourself the opportunity to make a choice. See if you can love yourself with a choice that serves you best – that casts a vote in favour of future you - most of the time.

Make Your Patterns And Paths Work For You

Humans are creatures of habit. Your brain is designed to shortcut activities that you repeat from day to day. This is a survival mechanism that allows you to get stuff done. Think about when you first learned to drive the car. How aware and conscious did you need to be about every step in the process. Putting your belt on, adjusting your mirrors, finding where to put the key, knowing where the knobs and dials and switches were, carefully steering and monitoring if you were in the lane correctly. Now think about that last time you left work and arrived home and you don't even remember a minute about the drive. Your eating patterns can be like that. Maybe some of the patterns you have are really positive? good? ones - Great! Do more of them. Maybe some of the patterns you have don't serve you at all anymore – Great! Now you know. As you get aware of your environment look for these patterns and then experiment with ways to break the chain. Where can you disrupt the pattern to open the opportunity to do it differently. Do you drive by the Tim Hortons on your way into work each day and automatically pull in for a coffee? And when you get a coffee, do you *always* get a muffin? Do you come in the front door from work put your bags down and go right to the fridge? Do you do your planning at the end of the day at the kitchen table and automatically pull something down from the cupboard on your way there? What if you took a different route that didn't take you past the Tim Hortons? What if you started storing your work bag in a room upstairs so you would go there first instead of the kitchen, or planned to change out of your work clothes first thing when you go home? What if you moved your planning space from the kitchen table to a desk or another space in the house? What changes can you make in your environment that disrupts unwanted patterns and paths and creates opportunity to create new ones that are in support of desired future you?

Set Up Your Kitchen

If you're going to eat better, you're going to spend time in your kitchen. So not only is it going to be more pleasant if you set things up well, it's also going to help you be there more and be more efficient when you are. Get curious about the placement of things in your kitchen. Are the cutting boards and knives in the area you'll be doing prep? Do you have the tools you need to make that prep smooth? Could rearranging some cupboards or investing in a good knife or cutting board shape the path? Would you enjoy some music while you are there or some pictures or art on the wall that make you smile? Is it time to replace the tattered throw mat in front of the kitchen sink? You get the idea.

Internal Environment

Your internal environment can be a little trickier to navigate, and the obstacles can be less obvious that the ones you can see around you with your eyes. One big difference between your external and internal environment is that some things in your external environment are out of your control to change, but your internal environment is totally your domain! When you become aware of the beliefs and thought patterns that serve you, and those that don't, you have an opportunity to change them. When you can get to a place that the voices in your head or the feelings in your body boost you instead of beat you down, you create and environment inside you that is safe for growth and change. It's about setting your internal environment to allow you to thrive and use all the gifts you have to become all you are meant to be.

Here is a tour of key aspects to focus in in your internal landscape:

Do What Matters To You

What matters to you? What's important to you? What are the things you believe make up a good life for you? A life the way you want to live it. Reflect on these questions. Record them in your Owner's Manual. These are your *values*. Take a minute to think if what you've written it's totally your own or if it might be jumbled up with others ideas of what's important in life. Now take a look at your calendar. Take a look at what you have scheduled and what you protect your time to do. How does the way you spend your days compare that to what you believe matters most? Where do they line-up? Where are they misaligned? As you work through your Owner's Manual and as you make choices in your day, get in the habit of checking in to see if the choices you're making, the principles you're following, and the actions you're taking align with your values. Do you believe you are honouring your values with your actions? Bring all the kindness and self-compassion you have as you explore this questions because with all the external noise that can get in your way, living your values is no small feat in today's world. You have experienced what misalignment feels like (I bet there's a good chance it was that feeling that got you here reading this book). Let that inspire action in you to try it a different way. Pick one small place to nudge something closer to what matters to you. Then do that again, and again, and again.

Choose Who You Will Be

Your identity is who you think you are. Who you believe yourself to be? I like to think of identity as being made up of a collection of smaller identities instead of one big solid lump.. Sure, there are overarching themes and interconnectedness about identity (linked to your values) but there can also be individuality and uniqueness in different places too. You identity as a professional, as a friend, as a child, as a parent, as a partner. If you're a task-oriented doer in your work life there's no reason you can't be free-floating take-it-as-it-comes-er on the weekend. Identities also don't have to be *either/or*, they can be *both* and you can bring all parts of yourself with you. Each one can function as part of the bigger identity but is also be small enough to adapt and change and grow in a way that aligns more closely with what matters to you. You don't have to overhaul the whole deal and feel like you have to leave behind your entire self in order to make room for new pieces of who you are. On the other hand, there are times that breaking up or deliberately killing a piece of your identity *is* necessary to make room for you to embrace a new one. Some identities cannot coexist just by nature. For instance, to become a non-smoker you can't identify as a smoker and as a non-smoker at the same time. The old part of you that was a smoker *has* to go. Some identities used to serve you but they don't any more. Turn your awareness to who you believe you are and how that causes you to show up in the world. How is that serving you now? Does that identity truly align with what matters to you now? Is time to try on something new?

Worth Is Not Attached To Weight

Girls Gone Strong posted this from Molly Galbraith and Jen Comas; "If you have a goal of losing weight in order to feel better, move better – or frankly for whatever reason you desire (#YourBodyYourBusiness) – I completely respect your choice. But I implore you remember that your worth is not attached to your weight, regardless of what that number is." That is worth reading twice.

It's time for a heart-to-heart about weight. Your weight does not define your worth –not your personal worth, not your professional worth. Nor does how you eat, or what you wear, or what job or house or car you have, or what you love or don't love to do. There is no such thing as having to *earn* your worth. "I know, Irene," you say. I know you know. But do you *really* know? Like, do you deep down in your soul believe that to be true?

When you do the work we do, it's easy to find yourself believing that your weight and your worth are in fact one in the same somedays. The truth is you have gifts you bring into this world that cannot possibly be measured by a scale. Ever. I'm not here to blow sunshine up your butt, but I am here to be outside eyes and nudge you to begin to see and believe that truth. You have a life to live. Your time flying around on this big blue sphere doesn't wait for you to lose weight. And it doesn't start once you've lost weight. It's here. Right now. Your life. Get on with that first. Include this as part of that life if you want. But live regardless. Tune your awareness up to what you believe you are worth in this life. What you believe you deserve. Get curious about where that comes from. Hold space for yourself as you explore this and bring your kindness and compassion as you do. If you discover there are some things here that need extra attention, get help. You deserve that, too.

You Can Cheat At Cards But Not At Eating

Think about the language you use as you talk about food. Cheat implies there is morality to eating – nothing good can come from that. Change the language and you change your mindset to serve you better. Sometimes you get to choose the worse choice and that is totally ok and totally normal and totally within the choices you are free to make as a grown up in this world. I wonder what would happen if you fully give yourself that permission to choose? Curiosity really helps here. Anytime you have a sense of judgment about yourself (or someone else), see what happens if you drop into curiosity. "Huh. Look at what I'm doing (or he or she is doing). Isn't that interesting. I wondering what that's about? I wonder what might be going on for me (him/her) right now?" Change from *cheat* to *choice* and give yourself permission to make any darn decision you want. You deserve that.

Rewrite Outdated Stories And Scripts

You have stories you tell yourself about yourself. Some of the stories have been with you a long time. The first stories you took on about your map of the world and your place in it came from your experiences as a child. You came to believe certain things to be true. As powerful as they can feel, the bottom line is they are stories. Stories that you hold authorship of, and you can choose to rewrite in any way you want at any time you choose. When you believe that to be true, it is both freeing and whole lotta scary. What it means is that you are essentially responsible for them. You are responsible for who you become and what you believe about the world. Employ your awareness, curiosity, and compassion about your stories. As always, you don't have to change anything. It's always your call. See which stories you tell yourself have served you and how. Do they still serve you now? Which stories may have served you in the past but no longer do? It's rarely all-or-nothing. Parts of the story may serve you while other parts do not. Tune in and decide if it's time to get out your red pen and edit a few lines or start a fresh page all together.

Let Worry Inspire Action

See if you can notice when you find yourself in your head, wondering and worrying about something that may or may not happen in the future. You can spend massive amount of emotional energy in the wonder and worry space and it's no fun. When you notice you're in that space, call it out and ask yourself, "Does this makes sense? Do these thoughts serve me? What kind of action does this worry inspire in me (if any) and what do I want to do about that?"

Navigating and shifting your internal environment takes patience and practice. It's common to have years of deeply ingrained negative self-talk or feelings or views or beliefs about yourself that get in the way of you making changes in your life. That get in the way of you showing up in the world as a more authentic version of you. Awareness and practice along with a healthy dose of self-compassion are key. Know that you are completely normal for having these things in the way of your progress right now. Also know it doesn't have to stay that way if you don't want it to. Tune in and gently begin to shift to kindness. Ask yourself, "How can I be kind to myself right now?" "What would this look like if I were caring for somebody else in this?" Chances are this way of relating to yourself will feel completely foreign and uncomfortable. Maybe way more "touchy-feely" that what feels ok for you. Be brave enough to do it anyway. When the day comes that you catch yourself automatically defaulting to kindness and self-compassion you'll think, "Huh. Isn't that curious."

Questions for Reflection - Environment

Start Here

What does my environment look like right now? What in my environment is serving me? What is getting in the way of my forward progress?

Get Curious

Get curious about the following things in your environment. Think about places you may be able to try something different.
Triggers – are there things around that trigger you? What would happen if you eliminated those or what would happen if you chose to change the trigger? If you chose to let pain or discomfort trigger reflection for you?
Patterns – what do you notice? Is there a way to disrupt the pattern you see?
Feeling links – do you notice specific feeling linked to specific behaviours?
People links – a specific behaviours linked to certain people or even places

Try Stuff

What easy low hanging fruit things can I change, now that I'm aware of them? Where are the bright spots? How can I do more of that? What obstacles can I clear to shape my path? What stories or thoughts or beliefs or identities are no longer serving me? How can I rewrite those?

Part IV:

Reclaim

Chapter 10:
Take Action – Turn Knowing into Doing

"Knowing what to do will not change your life."
- Mel Robbins

Once you have the foundations of your Owner's Manual, it's time to put it into action. Here are the fundamentals actions of change that I believe to be true based on my work with clients and my own experience.

Change Requires Doing And Experiencing

People change by doing and experiencing, not by knowing alone. Bring to mind a sport you've played or an instrument you learned or an activity you took part in. Imagine it's basketball and I arrived to a room full of people new to basketball, and I handed them each a huge book all about basketball. I sent them off with instructions to read the book and asked them to come back in four weeks. When they arrived, I hand them some running shoes and asked them to show me how to play. The whole scenario sounds absurd, right? Of course, it does. Yet this is essentially what you ask of yourself with eating (and also with personal development). You read all the stuff and can recite all the stuff, and then you read more stuff and expect yourself to just execute what you now know. You don't allow space and time to be new at that thing. No time for practice. No time for growth and development of the skills necessary to execute it. You expect you can just go, and then you are disappointed that it didn't work.

If you want to eat better and reap the benefits of that, you have to practice eating better. Plain and simple. Allow yourself time and space to build and hone skills. That requires experience – putting the reps in. I have good news for you! Each time you eat is an opportunity to practice. If you eat three times per day, seven days per week, fifty-two weeks per year, that is 1092 practice sessions per year. If you had that many basketball practices or piano lessons or chess matches each year, you certainly could make some pretty amazing progress if you showed up consistently, right? Well yes, but only if you showed up with the intention to practice and the belief that you could get better (that growth mindset thing again).

When you eat, you often just eat. What if you considered each time you eat a chance to practice doing it a little better? What if you stick with a small focus, like eating more slowly, and continued that practice each time you ate? How much progress do you think you could make in a week (twenty-one practices) or a month (147 practices)?

Focus On One Thing At A Time

Your chance of success greatly increased when you focus on one thing at a time. When you're trying to change a number of things at one time, your focus is divided. Divided focus is less effective. It makes sense, right? Your focus is spread so thin that you don't have a strong enough focus on any one thing to do it well. That is not a problem with you; it's a problem with the system. It is a poor environment to get better in – plain and simple. By pulling back and actually focusing on less, you end up being able to achieve more. Doing less is a path to doing more. If you'd like to read more on this topic, check out *The Power of Less* by Leo Babauta.

Here's a great time to check in with your expectations and what you know to be true about the process of change. Are you trying to fast track something that you know needs focus, time, and practice? Check in regularly on the number of things you're focusing on. Really check in. Play the honesty card here. "Do I believe I am upping my success by focusing on one thing at a time?" "What is my one thing today/this week?" Not one *category* that includes twenty things … one thing. Show yourself or an accountability partner or coach that you can do it consistently before you move onto the next thing.

If you are able to really focus in on the one thing you are doing, you are much more likely to build that one habit or skill more deeply and be able to incorporate it as a regular part of your life moving forward. When you're starting a change process and truly applying this principle, things are likely going to feel uncomfortable. Like its moving along a little more slowly than you would like. You're motivated, you're excited, and you just want your darn pants to fit already! Take a breath and remind yourself that less is more.

When You Can Just Do A Little, Do A Little

Doing something is better than doing nothing, no matter how small that something is. It's easy for *all-or-nothing* thinking to get in the way of what you really want because it prevents you from taking any action that isn't the biggest action. I can't eat the perfect meal I had planned, so I'll just have a burger and fries instead. I can't do my regular one-hour workout, so I won't do any workout at all. All-or-nothing thinking shows up over and over and over in your life. When you do life this way, you build your on-again off-again muscle and *that* becomes your default. Suppose instead of training that muscle, you trained your consistency muscle? You let consistency of action be your goal and become someone who will always take action in the direction of your goal – no matter how small. A huge opportunity really does exist in the space between all and nothing.

In each week, day, or moment, ask yourself, "Will I do a little or a do a lot?" Whichever answer you choose; you are doing *something*. When you practice *always-something* thinking, you end up taking consistent action towards your goal. Consistency over time is where the magic of change is. The book *The Slight Edge* by Jeff Olson explains this concept brilliantly. He explains that the slight edge is a way of thinking about all the choices you make and actions you take in a day. Each action, no matter how big or small, is a step toward or away from what you want – there is no neutral. Over time, the side that gets more votes is where you will end up.

There is a lot of room between all and nothing.

When you can just do a little, do a little. When you can do a lot, do a lot. Allow the level and intensity of your effort to ebb and flow with the demands of life. Think about each area of your life as a dial that can be turned up or turned down - but not turned off (e.g. family, career, personal health, and fitness). In any given period of time, you are adjusting dials up and down as needed; when demands in one area dial up, you dial another area down. If you have a day or week where demands in other areas are less and you can dial up efforts elsewhere (say in your fitness and nutrition), do it! Celebrate that you were able to hit the gym an extra time this week or prepared and froze a batch of chili one day. Just because you can't commit to doing it every week, doesn't mean you can't do it *this* time. If you let the fact that you can't do something from now until forever get in the way of you doing it at all, you are missing an opportunity to log some extra progress towards your desired version of future you. Make a practice of casting extra votes in that direction whenever you get the chance.

In bringing the actions in your Owner's Manual to life, practice noticing when you fall into all-or-nothing thinking, and move yourself towards always something thinking instead.

Principles For Taking Action

Here are ten strategies to help you take consistent action. Some of them are slightly different versions of the same thing, but you may find one speaks to you more than another. You know the system now; try them on and see which ones work for you, and then do more of that.

Make consistency of action the goal

Instead making the outcome you want your goal (like a specific weight), make taking consistent actions that move you towards that goal the goal. If you can nail the consistency of your actions, you will make fast progress towards your end goal.

Go all in on the thing you are doing

As you know by now, language matters for me. How you ask yourself something can make all the difference in how you are able to execute it (if at all). What I'm talking about here could be called *being present* or being *in the moment*. If that language work for you, fantastic – do that. The idea of being present ties in closely with awareness (you touched on this in Chapter 4), but they are a little different. Awareness is paying attention. Being present is *going all in* on the one thing you are doing right now. Awareness naturally comes when you go *all in*, but it is possible to be aware without being all in. Dividing your awareness to multiple things at the same time is easy to do in a multi-tasking culture full of distraction. When you say to yourself, "Go all in on this now," you are either all in or you aren't. You can't be *half* all in.

Go all in on your eating when you are eating. Go all in on the conversation with the person you are talking to. Go all in on doing the dishes. Go all in on the work you are doing. Go all in on reading this book.

See how it works. It's a guiding magical statement that directs you to focus on the one thing that is in front of you right now. And it brings to your awareness when you have wandered. As soon as you feel the wander, you will know you're not all in and can kindly pull yourself back.

In the absence of clarity, take action

There were times I got stuck waiting to have a clear goal or perfect plan. Like I couldn't start until I knew exactly where I was headed. Not having a clear goal ended up being a reason not to start. I could convince myself that I was *working* on this problem because I was working on figuring out my goal, even though I was taking *no* real action in the direction of desired future me. So, when I don't have a clear goal, I live by this quote from Philip McKernnan, one of my coaches, "In the absence of clarity take action."

I can do something that I know is in the general direction of where I'm headed while I'm waiting to figure out my specific goal. I can stop doing something that I know is not part of where I'm headed, while I'm waiting to clarify my goal.

For example, if I don't have a specific fitness goal I'm clear on, I know whatever that goal is won't include *no* exercise. I can put my running shoes on and go for a run even though I don't know *exactly* how running fits into some larger fitness goal.

Tools For Taking Action

Focus on the *starting* part

If you get stuck not starting, then lower the threshold to start. Once you start, there is a good chance you will continue. When I was first beginning to work on my nutrition business in a meaningful way, I found myself not doing the work I wanted to do. It was important to me – really important – but the *starting* part was getting in the way. My brain would play games with me as I looked at the long list of things I wanted to be working on but wasn't. So I wouldn't do *anything*. Or I would do the less hard, less important stuff. I reached out to the coach I was working with at the time, Craig Ballantyne, and told him I was stuck. He said this, "Can you get up fifteen minutes earlier and work on your business – *one* thing (not social media related) that is important to your business?" Of course I could do that. What do you think happened? You got it. Each day, I got the fifteen minutes in and most days, I would work for an hour or more on the important stuff (like writing this book) just because I started. Have you ever gotten to the gym or prepared a great meal full of green-light food for yourself and said, "Gee. I wish I didn't do that." Right. Starting is sometimes all we need to do what we intend to do. Lower the threshold so you can get an "Oh yeah, I can do that." Aim for a 9/10; you can get it done. Do that. Start there, and see what happens.

Make time

If it matters, it deserves space on your calendar. If it doesn't get on your calendar, it won't get done. Your actions are your values playing out in your daily life. Do they line up for you right now? If eating really matters to you, show it in your actions. If time with your family really matters, show it in your actions. Dedicate time to it. Your human brain makes this process way more complicated than it needs to be. It is so easy to over think but it doesn't need to be complicated. Sure, things get in the way of executing *sometimes*, but if your overriding pattern points in a direction away from your values, it is time to revisit what *really* matters to *you* and reset your actions to align. Open your calendar right now. What things are on there that you won't skip or move? What things are the first things to get moved? Get curious. What is it about each of those things that has you execute them differently? Your calendar is a living snap shot of where you place your focus and energy. What is one small change you could make today to nudge your calendar more in alignment with what matters to you?

Automate

Once you know what works, you can eliminate the number of decisions you have to make in a day by setting up systems and routines that essentially make the decisions for you.

When you find things that work for you, think about how you can automate or create routines around as many of those tasks as you can. Where can you tag desired actions to other behaviors you're already doing (drink a glass of water first thing on waking in the morning)? Can you set your environment up to support a sequence of steps that get you to take an action that matters for you (have the blender and non-perishable ingredients out and ready on the counter for your shake in the morning). Commit to practice a specific routine for at least two weeks of time to begin to groove the habit (like a bedtime routine). If you eat so much better with a few meals prepped and ready, automate some meal prep as part of your regular Sunday routine. Go back through your Owner's Manual. Look at what worked for you – especially those habits that you know to be key – and ask yourself, "How can I automate this or pieces of this?"

Set up Guardrails

Guardrails. You know the little fence-like things along the road or the highway the keep you from driving your car off the cliff? Or the little bumper bars that pop up in bowling so you don't get a gutter ball like every time (speaking for a friend)? Look at your Owner's Manual and think about where you tend to drive off the road. How can you put some guardrails up there? Some guidelines you will lovingly put in place for yourself to keep you safe on the path to desired future you?

BAMs

BAM stands for Bare A** Minimums. These are the things you commit to doing each day or week as a minimum. If ten on the dial is you being a nutrition super star and zero is you making no deliberate effort to look after your nutrition at all, your BAM is *one* on the dial. The absolute smallest action you will continue to take no matter what. This is your plan to *stay in the game* and continue making votes in favor of you. Take one tiny action in the direction of your goals, even if the rest of your day is like a dumpster fire. This is your commitment to you, to show up for you, and to train your always-something (versus all-or-nothing) muscle.

Your BAMs are woven into your identity that you are a person whose dial for x does not go lower than y. Perhaps your BAM for vegetables is one per day, which means even on a day the you know what totally hits the fan in the worst kind of way, you will find a way to get at least one vegetable in. Maybe your BAM for exercise is a ten-minute body weight workout that you hammer out no matter what – even if that is push-ups and air squats beside your bed in the morning. BAMs keep you taking actions in the direction of your goals no matter what. You continue to practice your consistency muscle and stay out of all-or-nothing thinking because no matter what, you can count on yourself to do your BAMs.

Do the imperfect thing

This has got to be one of my favorite ways to get myself going. If you have a perfectionist part of you, you may love this one too. Ask yourself, "How can I do an imperfect version of the perfect thing right now?" You will be amazed how much fast action this can inspire in you and how good it can feel to do something versus holding out until you can only do the perfect version. This will feel silly and even at times meaningless at first, but I assure you it's not. Once you get in the swing of doing the imperfect thing, it can actually become a fun little game. Here are some examples:

- Imperfect weekly veggie prep? Wash and cut three carrots.
- Imperfect one hour workout? Ten minute walk or ten jumping jacks right now.
- Imperfect kitchen clean up? Wash five dishes.

Make a vote in favor of you

You've heard me use this one again and again throughout the book. This is my go-to check in with myself. "How can I make a vote in favor of me right now?" "What would a vote in favor of me look like in this situation?" In a clean poll between two candidates (let's imagine in kindergarten class versus national politics), the math is simple, the more votes one gets the more likely they are to win. Consider your days a contest between the desired version of future you and the less desired version of future you. Some version of you will win. Its up to current you to decide which one that will be by casting votes in favor of the one you want most. Every action you take is a vote in favor of one of them, there is no neutral vote. Cast votes in favor of desired future you anywhere and everywhere you can. You don't need a plan or system for voting. You just get to cast and cast and cast. And the outcome will take care of itself.

Chapter 11:

Steer Dynamically - Navigate Common Obstacles

"I see your pain, and it's big.
I also see your courage, and it's bigger.
You can do hard things."
- Glennon Doyle

Even if you follow this formula and execute the steps here well, you will bump up against obstacles. Here are three you are likely to encounter: the grind, others, and your old self. I'm giving you a heads up to keep a look out for these. When they do come up for you, you want to know. Step into the reality of it and you will be in a better mindset, "Ah! Here's that thing that I was expecting. I go this."

How To Get Through The Grind

Chances are you're feeling pretty motivated right now. You've got this book, a plan to follow and you're pumped and ready for action. Celebrate that and enjoy the rush of wanting to get started. While you're here in that pumped up space, let's talk about what to do when that feeling fades. Because it will. When your reality feels less pumped up and more like a grind you *want* to see that and step into it.

When you hit the grind, don't wait for motivation to take action. Take action to spark motivation. It seems like the opposite of what we've been taught but the reality is if you wait to do the things that matter until you *feel* like it, they're never going to get done. Be the creator and the master of your own motivation and you won't ever have to wait for it again.

Here are some tools to use to help you through the grind:

Reboot

Go back to the beginning of the book and begin again. Reignite your beginner and growth mindset. Revisit your values and what matters to you and what trade-offs you're willing to make to create your best life possible.

5-4-3-2-1

Mel Robbin's 5 Second Rule has helped me start again in places I've felt stuck more times than I can count. The practice is so simple but super powerful. When you have a thought about an action to take, count down from *five* and when you hit *one* - you go! In those five seconds you boost yourself into action mode. 5-4-3-2-1 go! You can check out her Ted Talk explaining it here https://youtu.be/Lp7E973zozc

After I __. Then I'll ___.

This little formula strings two actions together and helps build behaviors in a simple yet powerful way. It is focused on action and can be the nudge you need to move through the grind, one step at a time, even when you don't feel like it. This strategy comes from BJ

Fogg, the creator of Tiny Habits. You can check out more about this here https://youtu.be/AdKUJxjn-R8

Celebrate

Yes celebrate. The tiniest of little things. Celebrate them all. A little fist pump. A little (or a big), "Yaaassss! I did that!" or an, "Ooooh yah!". Your brain loves a little rush and celebration so get it working for you. Each time you take an action in the direction of desired future you, or follow through on a promise you made to yourself, or feel scared and do it anyway, or show up for yourself, or make a vote in favor of you, celebrate it. (Yess! I just finished that paragraph!)

When Others Seem To Sabotage Your Efforts

The people in your life that love you, love you. But because you are ready to change, does not mean they are ready to change, and it also does not mean they are ready for you to change. It's easy to get caught off guard and discouraged and thrown for a bit of a spin when the people around you (especially the ones that matter most to you) seem to sabotage the efforts you're making to create a better life for yourself. The reality is, it has absolutely nothing to do with you and everything to do with their stuff and where they are and what they are ready or not ready to do. Seeing your bravery to go after what matters to you, can bring up all kinds of stuff for them (often painful stuff). Bring your curiosity and compassion for them but also bring your awareness, curiosity, and compassion for yourself and how they are choosing to act and respond is impacting you. They may need some space for a while to adjust to who you are now. It's also cue for you to think about what really matters most to you and how the people in your life fit into that. Before you react, think about how their reaction might make sense. They don't have a window to the change that's going on inside you. They only experience that the "you" they used to know is not the same. Your talk about changing things and getting better may be felt as harsh judgment on them as they continue doing the same things the two of you used to do together that the new (better) you, no longer does. You used to split bottles of wine, crush bags of chips, and binge watch Netflix. Now the new you is drinking water, portioning chips onto a plate or crunching veggies, and talking about the last documentary you saw. Makes sense?

Ask yourself, "If I were in their shoes, is it possible that I might feel or believe what they do?" At the same time that you want to come at this with compassion, you also want to be mindful of what matters to you and all the energy and effort you have put into getting in alignment yourself. Try having open and honest conversation and see if they can share in excitement for you. If they can't it certainly can be difficult (and painful) but consider what may be best for you. Talk about it with someone who gets where you are. Open conversation and time for them to get to know you as you are now are a great approach to take. One of the best strategies to help you navigate this, is to just know it's coming and call it out when it does.

When Your Old Self Gets In Your Way

Sometimes it's not others that get in your way, but pieces of old you that hang on strong. Bring your awareness, curiosity and self-compassion. Where does old you show up the strongest? What do you think that might be about? It's often about identity and stories. Old identities that once served you that don't serve you anymore. The good news is you can rewrite these. Some stories and piece of you can shift and evolve to continue to serve you. Some stories and pieces of you have to completely die for the new parts of you to come to life. A powerful exercise is to write a breakup letter to your old self. It can be soft and an easy let down thanking *Old You* for the ways he/she used to help you and letting him/her know it is time for new you to move on. It can be a hard crash and burn heavy metal break up that sends Old You packing (don't let the door hit you on the way out!) Write it down: Dear Old Me, ... Connect with all these pieces of you. When you are feeling stuck along your journey, see if there is another part that is ready to go too. And do it again.

Chapter 12:
Own It – You Got This

"Sometimes the strength within you is not a big fiery flame for all to see. It is just a tiny spark that whispers ever so softly, 'you got this, keep going.'"

- Unknown

Congratulations, you made it! Remember that celebration thing from the last chapter? Yup. Take a moment to do that now (*Woo Hoo!*) Let's recap:

Part I: Reality

You took the brave move of stepping into *your* reality which includes that fact that you are human and therefore get to navigate the same inconveniences of being human as everyone else does (again, welcome to the club). You learned that misaligned expectations, ownership, and actions show up again and again and that placing some focus on resetting these is time well spent in the interest of change. You decided that leaning into discomfort and difficult things is worth it to make the change you want in your life, and that you deserve to get help along the way as you need it. You learned about creating your Owner's Manual as a tool to capture what you discover in this process and as a way to create a living set of handling instructions to follow that are specific to your body, your life, and what work's best for you.

Part II: Reboot

Here you tapped into your beginner and growth mindsets to start where you are, check in with your expectations, and reboot them in places they are no longer serving you. You learned about the gap and the tension between where you *are* and where you think you *should be* and how you can close that gap both by changing where you are and by changing expectations around where you think you should be.

Next, you learned how dropping into curiosity, instead of judgment, and brining awareness and self-compassion to all you do can not only help you through this but can change the entire way experience life. You learned tools to build your awareness, curiosity, and self-compassion skills and strategies that will help you remember to practice.

Awareness opens the possibility and opportunity for meaningful change. It creates space for you to try stuff. You learned principles and strategies for experimenting and evaluating in ways that will allow you to figure out what works best for you.

Part III: Reset

You brought those newly learned skills and principles to lay the groundwork for your own reset. First you focused your lens on basics of eating better using the five steps to reset:

Step 1: Why: Know why you're eating
Step 2: How: Slow down and leave some room
Step 3: Where: Eat where you eat best
Step 4: What: Get your basic plate in shape

Step 5: When: Eat when you are hungry

You then moved on to build the movement and sleep sections of your Owner's Manual. And finally, you were reminded of the huge importance both your internal and external environments have on the choices that you make. You now have tools and strategies to create the right environment in your head and around you to support your desired future you.

In Part IV: Reclaim

You brought it all together with strategies to get consistent and persistent no matter what life throws your way. You know some of the common roadblocks that may present themselves as you get to the grind stage and your motivation wanes.

I celebrate you for being brave enough to be here because I know from my own journey it is not an easy thing to do. I also know from my own journey that being brave enough to reach out can lead you down a path you've never expected. I'm excited to hear where your path leads.

When you get curious, you will discover a whole lot about yourself and the ways you interact with the world around you. The ways you 'do life' so to speak. Some of what you learn about yourself will surprise and even delight you. Some of what you learn will leave you feeling defeated and stuck (if you let it).

My next challenge for you is to begin to entertain the idea that you're exactly where you are meant to be. How would you show up if you believed that? If you knew what you needed right now, was right here. That it's ok to be the expert and at the same time be brave enough to be the client. To know all the things and start at the beginning, anyhow. To be afraid and do it, anyway. To show up for yourself and do something when you don't feel like doing anything at all.

You are going to fail; yes, you will fail. Everyone does at some point because figuring this out will require you to try stuff and get it wrong to know what doesn't work and try stuff and get it right to know what does. Both are not only likely but essential. There is no growth in comfort. And life won't pause while you are in the grind. Not because you are doomed somehow but because you are human.

My wish for you is that you treat your body like it belongs to someone you love and you care for yourself like someone you are responsible for caring for. When you believe you deserve to be cared for that way, things change. Pause and think about that for a minute … *like someone you are responsible for caring for*. Have you ever cared for a child or a fur baby (like how I grouped them together)? You are *responsible* for caring for them. They are counting on you with their life. You deliver. You feed them the well. You limit their candy and table scraps (ok, food off the car floor is fair game). You make sure they get outside for fresh air and exercise each day. You make sure they get sleep. You love them with kind words and hugs and laughs and play and the things that bring them joy.

You deserve that, too. All of it. You are worth it. If that just made you squirm in your seat, don't worry, I'll continue to say it for you – until you're able to consistently say it out loud yourself (and accept it as truth). You can borrow from me for as long as you need.

You are worth it.

Everybody has B.S. in their life. Everyone. All the time. It is called being human. Who do you want to be despite the fact that you are dealing a ridiculous number of things? If you wanted to let those things stop you, you wouldn't be here. Those things are not your choice but being here is. And you, my friend, are here. And I'm certainly glad you are.

Let's do this. I'm rooting for you. xo

Further Reading

Tiny Beautiful Things by Cheryl Strayed
*You are a Bada*** by Jen Sincero
The 5 Second Rule by Mel Robbins
The Slight Edge by Jeff Olson
Principles by Ray Dalio
The Power of Less by Leo Babauta
Atomic Habits by James Clear

Acknowledgments

My children Daphne Lacey and Hugh bring sparks of joy to my days and the warmth from them flowed into these pages. Thank you for your cuddles, and your smiles, and your laughs as I wrote. Thanks for being patient with piles of paper, last minute (but healthy) meals, and the hours of time you watched me typing at my desk (I'm sorry to say this finished book means there may be less screen time for you moving forward). Thank you for sharing what is in your hearts with me and for accepting and loving me for what is in mine. For you I embrace the dark and the light that life has to offer to show you that it can be done and that it is possible to build your days around what matters most to you. Thank you to Andrew for supporting my book writing journey with generosity of time, resources, and heart.

Thank you to my Mum, Dad and Ce, sisters Jenn and Julia, and my extended family for the role you played in getting me here. I love you all with my whole heart. Special thanks to my Opa, Nikolaus Zeis (your name is now in my book) for babysitting, playing chauffeur, and coming each week to make a delicious meal (including blaukraut and knoodle) for us while I wrote. Ich liebe dich.

Thank you to friends, old and new, for showing up again and again in exactly the way I needed, at exactly the right moment. Every one of your texts, calls, messages, and visits lifted me in a way more powerful than you could know. Every boost from each of you made this possible.

Love and thanks to Snydes, Shannon and my field hockey family for the regular check ins, straight talk when I needed it, and unwavering belief in me through this. I know you ladies (I use that term loosely) have my back.

Lisa Stamper, I am grateful for the contagious squeals of joy and excitement that came out of you as I shared stories about my journey writing this book (a can hear them now). Thank you for the light you brought me through this.

Dev Chengkalath my friend, you've been a rock in so many ways on this book writing journey - thank you with all of me (MBE or bust). Thanks to Mike Gillespie for the check-ins and laughs and sharing your belief in this project and excitement for me - it's go time! To GL Pascale, it's fitting that we met the day the seed was planted for this book. Thanks for seeing great things in me from that moment and continuing to challenge me - I could hear your voice in my head on the days I needed it (11 out of 10). Thank you to Allison Graham for the impromptu brainstorm phone sessions that ended up being pivot points in the direction of this book.

Thank you to Lauren Hamelin, the Loblaw Dietitian team, and colleagues at Zehrs Stanley Park and Glenridge for your support and enthusiasm as I made an unexpected shift to write.

Thanks to John Berardi, Krista Scott-Dixon and the whole Precision Nutrition crew for seeing the value in fostering the community of amazing coaches you do and giving so generously of your wisdom and time. Connecting and finding a home there was the beginning of the journey that brought me here.

To the Author Incubator team and the other authors I have connected with through this, what an incredible gift you have all been at this time in my life. Thank you to Moriah for your patience and deep knowing I would get this done. Thank you to Angela Lauria for seeing what you see in me, knowing I can handle what I need to hear, and loving me enough to tell me.

Thank you to the Morgan James Publishing Team: David Hancock, CEO & Founder; my Author Relations Manager, Bonnie Rauch; and special thanks to Jim Howard, Bethany Marshall, and Nickcole Watkins.

Last but certainly not least, thank you to the professionals, coaches, and mentors who have changed my life in incredible ways and who's words and lessons fueled and fill these pages. Life continues to hand me the teachers I need in sometimes the most unexpected ways … for this book special thanks goes to these ones: Pam Ruhland, Jay Bonn, Denise Allen, Philip McKernan, Craig Ballantyne, Colin Lake, Edith Townsend, and Dr. Andrew Ekblad - thank you all for all the things.

Thank You

Thank you for reading *Eat Like You Teach* and for joining me in *experiencing* your way through the stuff of life. It sure can be a *windows-down-volume-up* kind of ride and company along the way makes it a whole lot better!

I celebrate you for your strength and courage. For being brave enough to build the life that matters most to you. I celebrate you for showing up each day in whatever way you can, and for each and every vote you make in favor of you. *Yessss!*

From the bottom of my heart, I'm honored to have been a part of this piece of your story. I'd love to hear from you! Pop over to www.irenepace.ca and tell me one vote you made in favor of *you* today (so I can celebrate with you!)

I'm rooting for you. xo

About the Author

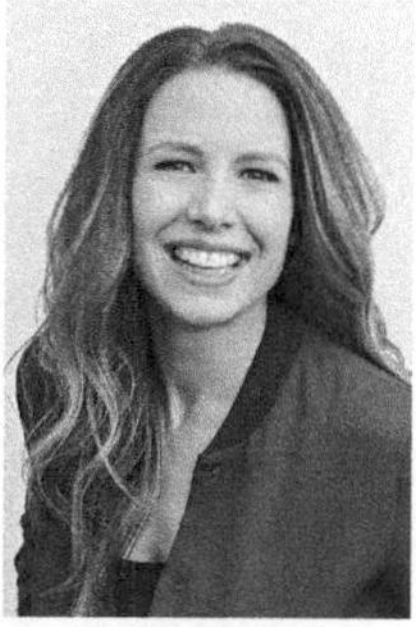

Irene Pace is a Registered Dietitian, coach, and speaker with over 15 years of experience helping people like you make the changes that matter most. With her confident, easy style, she'll empower you to see and leverage the skills you already have to improve your eating, your body, and your life.

From advanced clinical work at a lead trauma hospital to coaching hundreds of women online with world-class nutrition company *Precision Nutrition,* Irene's unique cross-industry experience shines through in her simple yet effective, practical approach. She cuts through the obstacles and confusion holding you back, helping you shape a clear path to your success.

With her upcoming book, *Eat Like You Teach: How to Reset Your Weight and Reclaim Your Life*, Irene is excited to dedicate her to time to coaching coaches, business leaders, and other high performers just like you who need a reset to get their eating and their weight back on track.

Website: www.irenepace.ca

Email: irene@irenepace.ca

Facebook: www.facebook.com/irene.pace

IG: @irenepace.rd

Printed in the USA
CPSIA information can be obtained
at www.ICGtesting.com
JSHW082344140824
68134JS00020B/1861

9 781642 796896